A Nurse in Time

For Elizabeth, Zoe,
Robert and Madeleine

A Nurse in Time

My Life as a Trainee Nurse in the 1930s

EVELYN PRENTIS

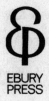

EBURY
PRESS

7 9 10 8

This edition published 2011 by Ebury Press, an imprint of
Ebury Publishing
A Random House Group company
First published in 1977 by Hutchinson & Co (Publishers) Ltd

The Random House Group Limited Reg. No. 954009

Addresses for companies within the Random House Group can be
found at www.randomhouse.co.uk

A CIP catalogue record for this book is available
from the British Library

The Random House Group Limited supports The Forest Stewardship
Council (FSC), the leading international forest certification organisa-
tion. All our titles that are printed on Greenpeace approved FSC
certified paper carry the FSC logo. Our paper procurement policy
can be found at www.rbooks.co.uk/environment

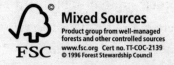

Mixed Sources
Product group from well-managed
forests and other controlled sources
www.fsc.org   Cert no. TT-COC-2139
© 1996 Forest Stewardship Council
FSC

Printed in the UK by CPI Cox & Wyman, Reading, RG1 8EX

ISBN 9780091941352

To buy books by your favourite authors and register for offers visit
www.rbooks.co.uk

Chapter One

IT MUST BE stressed from the start that I was not a born nurse. Not every girl is. Not every nurse is either, however wholeheartedly she may throw herself into the project once she gets going. Born nurses can be easily recognized. They have a little something the others haven't got which never seems to desert them however desperate the circumstances may become. They are to be envied.

Mothers of born nurses are just as easily picked out. They spend hours recalling the times their baby daughters sat about in corners playing at doctors and nurses, bandaging up their injured dollies and making poorly teddy bears better. I did none of these things. I never laid a bandage on a doll in my life.

The idea that I should be a nurse was entirely my mother's. It came to her one afternoon while she was in the middle of making the bread. She always made the bread on Friday afternoon. She washed, mangled and ironed on Monday, getting it all done down to the last handkerchief before she went to bed whatever the weather. If the trumpet had sounded on a Monday whoever was blowing it would have had to wait until the last bit of ironing had been folded and laid across the clothes horse to air. She did a bit to the bedrooms on Tuesday which took up most of the day.

On Wednesday she scrubbed, scoured and polished, and all with her bare hands as she masochistically boasted, every nook, plane and cranny in the house, taking in the bits that had been glossed over on Tuesday. And on Thursday, just in case anything had managed to escape her scrubbing brush and elbow grease, she did it all over again: but this time with greater vigour because on Friday the dust was allowed to settle and the house went to rack and ruin while she got on with the baking. The baking, like the bedrooms, took up most of the day.

As well as bread, vast quantities of pies, cakes and pasties were made on Fridays. My father liked his 'stuff' good and wholesome, and well burnt round the edges, and that was how we usually got it. Our oven could be a bit fierce sometimes according to which way the wind was blowing and the quality of the coal we happened to be using. On the other hand if it felt out of sorts for some reason or another, the pastry could come out as pallid as it was when it went in but a good deal harder. Like many other things where we lived, baking days were fraught with hazards.

The question of my career had cropped up yet again at school that afternoon. It had occupied my headmistress on and off for a long time.

'You will have to talk to your mother about it when you get home,' she had said nastily, among a lot of other nasty things. 'You must tell her that you have made up your mind to be a teacher.' I hadn't, she had. In spite of her brainwashing I wasn't convinced. All I was convinced about was that she wanted me out, and fast. This was understandable, I suppose. I was already seventeen and a well-built girl. The sixth form was bulging with girls who were seventeen and well built. She was probably getting desperate for space.

Whatever her reasons, she had made her point. She had finally persuaded me that the time had come for me to tell my mother that I wanted to be a teacher and the prospect was a daunting one. Nobody told my mother anything, least of all me. 'If there's any telling to be done round here I'll be the one to do it,' was a warning I had heard too often to take lightly. I expected no enthusiasm from her over my plans for the future and I got none. Her response was short, sharp and decisive. 'Rubbish,' she said and got on with the bread while I stood about nervously, waiting for more.

Just when it began to seem there was no more to come she wiped her hands on a flour bag, brushed a stray hair off her face and looked at me.

'I've been giving it a bit of thought,' she said, frowning. I don't reckon much on the idea of you being a teacher. It costs money to go to them training colleges and money doesn't grow on trees in this house. You'd be a lot better off being a nurse, you'd get paid right from the start and your food as well. As well as which,' she added, turning back to the dough, 'nursing's more ladylike,' and that clinched it for all of us.

Being ladylike was something my mother set great store by. She had spent a lot of time and trouble trying to turn me into a lady. That the project was doomed from the start was no fault of hers. I was simply never the right material for it. I resented the restrictions that being ladylike put upon me. I resented being robbed of so many pleasures in life. Simple pleasures like going potato picking in the holidays. All my cousins went potato picking and most of my friends as well and were able to earn themselves a tidy income at it, but my mother said it was common and kept me at home which not only got me a reputation in the village for being stuck-up but meant that I was always short of money. I was also short of excitement, and at least going potato picking might have given me more scope.

The biggest thrill we ever had in the village was when Lydia, the girl who slaved for the village schoolmistress, had sat down one night on a cracked chamber-pot and it had broken beneath her, causing indescribable and lasting injuries. Poor Lydia would never be the same again, or so I heard my mother telling my father when she got back from rendering first aid. They exchanged meaningful looks then glanced across at me and changed the subject. The reason my mother had been sent for in a hurry was because she was the only person in the village who knew anything about first aid. She had followed the doctor and helped him with his maternity cases until she married my father and became a farmer's wife, after which she concentrated her nursing skills on rearing sick pigs and bringing premature calves and lambs into the world. Except when there was an emergency like Lydia.

When the dough that my mother was working on had become as pliant beneath her firm hand as I was, she spoke again.

'Right,' she said, giving the pallid mass a final slap, 'that's all settled then, you can go and be a nurse. As soon as we've got the sugar beet off I'll see about getting you off.' Getting the sugar beet off was of paramount importance. Next to the pigs it was our main source of income and nothing was allowed to hinder its dispatch as the factory kept us to a tight schedule. But at least it was nice to know that my future was settled, and with a minimum of fuss and bother to anyone.

My mother wiped the flour from her fingers, put a clean tea-towel over the dough and set it in front of the fire to rise. She asked for no opinions from me on the career she had so arbitrarily chosen for me and I knew better than to offer any. To this day I seldom offer opinions unless I am invited to, and even then I like to be sure they will please everybody before I offer them. This can cause a lot of confusion among my friends and among my enemies as well. None of them is ever quite sure whose side I am on.

My mother's authority over me was absolute. When she said 'No', which was often, it was loud and clear and not open to question. She never felt called upon to explain an action or defend a decision. It was enough that she had said a thing to make it law. Her method of bringing up children was simple and straightforward. It was based on a few rules which she applied consistently and unflaggingly. Phrases like 'Children should be seen and not heard', 'Spare the rod and spoil the child' and other unarguable maxims were graffiti which were daily scrawled indelibly on my mind. If ever I showed signs of rebellion, which I seldom did – knowing better – I was sharply reminded of my place in the hierarchy of the family, often with the help of the nearest blunt instrument. She never confused me with indecision and we both knew exactly where we stood, with her firmly on top, and that was the way through use that I liked things to be.

Once my mother had made up her mind that I was going to be a nurse and had weighed up the advantages, she wasted no time in worrying about any possible disadvantages there might have been. That I was in no way cut out to be a nurse was no valid reason for me not becoming one. There had to be a more tangible excuse than that and nobody could find one.

I had had a 'good' education, which meant that I had bluffed my way through the scholarship when I was eleven. This entitled me to go to the girls' high school nine miles away where I spent the next six years battling to keep up with the fee-paying pupils. Academically this was not too difficult.

At the end of six years at the high school I had managed to pick up one or two of the nastier habits of the rich and enough of their accent to make me a laughing stock among my cousins and the friends of my village school days who had long since decided that I was nowt but a stuck-up thing and not worth bothering about, but I was still unable to grasp the finer points of relaxed eating which made me equally vulnerable during school dinners. These were referred to as 'lunch' by the rich girls. Lunch in our house was the light snack of bread and cheese, a slice or two of currant cake and a jam pasty that my father took with him when he went to work. He ate it round about ten o'clock in the morning sitting beneath a hedge on fine days, or standing with a sack wrapped round his legs to keep the wet out if it was raining. He cut the food into manageable chunks with the same clasp knife he used for cutting up his tobacco and he drank cold tea from a stone bottle. The birds gathered round him squabbling and queue jumping over their share of the crumbs he threw down for them.

The art of relaxed eating was something my mother had never taught me. Eating was a very serious matter in our house and not something to be undertaken lightly. She was strict about manners, especially about table manners. Not only was I not allowed to talk while I was eating but the least sound to escape my lips through chewing or swallowing was rewarded with a clout, gentle or sharp depending on her prevailing mood, and a sharp reminder to watch my manners in future or there would be more where that one came from. The noise some of those fee-paying girls made while they were eating whatever it was they called it would have destroyed my mother's faith in the ruling classes.

Being the woman she was, choosing a career for me had given my mother no more headaches than bringing me up had. Both responsibilities were shouldered with the same single-minded purposefulness. By a process of elimination, got through while she was kneading the dough, teaching would have been out from the start. The fact that my headmistress had decreed that I should be a teacher was enough, without any other consideration, to ensure that I never became one. My mother was not the sort of woman to be influenced by what others told her; she preferred to make her own decisions.

Chapter Two

WHEN THE LAST of the sugar beet had been dispatched to the factory and there was nothing more urgent to demand my mother's attentions she turned them to getting me off her hands. Once started she was fired with enthusiasm and suddenly seemed as anxious to see the back of me as my headmistress had been. She threw herself into the job of finding a place for me with all the zeal and much of the cunning of a woman launching her debutante daughter into society.

We were living on a smallholding in a remote and windswept part of Lincolnshire. Our house stood at the end of a long and permanently muddy cart-track. It was supported on one side by two blasted oak trees and on the other by an ancient monument we laughingly called a barn. Immediately next to the kitchen door was a large and odorous pigsty. There was no other habitation within sight of us and nothing to relieve the monotony of the landscape except the London Midland and Scottish railway which ran along the bottom of the garden to the detriment of the plaster on the bedroom ceilings.

Also at the bottom of the garden was the lavatory, or the closet as my father called it, though it bore no resemblance whatever to the American interpretation of the word. It was a rackety wooden building separated from the house by a rat-infested stream. If I happened to be sitting in there when a train rumbled past, the passengers and footplatemen made a point of looking across and waving to me. This courtesy had been made possible when the door fell off its hinges. My father never seemed to get round to nailing it back on again and it stood to the end of time propping up the water butt.

'Round the back' as my mother liked the lavatory to be called was definitely a summer place. In the summertime purple willowherb, honesty and fresh green stinging nettles grew in rich profusion round the open doorway, forcing their way through the floor boards and into the cracks of the seat, thus making it necessary to exercise extreme caution before sitting down. But in the winter it was bleak and dreary, only to be visited in times of desperate need and after the most detailed preparations had been made for the journey. When the weather was bad we never ventured round the back unless we were suitably clad in top-coat, gloves, scarf and a woolly hat. If it was raining we wore our wellingtons and took an umbrella with us. After dark it was necessary to carry a hurricane lamp to see our way safely past the stream. One false step and we were in it up to our knees, churning the mud and sending the rats scurrying in all directions.

Inside the rackety little shack there was a seating arrangement placed conveniently above a zinc bucket. The bucket had to be emptied once a week, or twice if we had visitors or a gastric disturbance. My father always emptied it on Saturday night just before he had his bath. My mother made him bath last.

The great drawback of our lavatory was that it only accommodated one person at a time. An aunt of mine up in the village had a lavatory that could seat three people in comfort. The holes were graduated in size: small, medium and large. I never saw it filled to capacity but there was a richness about it that was lacking in ours. The woodwork was of solid mahogany and there was always a strip of coconut matting down on the floor. My mother used to call this 'showing off', but I liked it and thought it made the place look nice and cosy.

As well as guiding our feet past the pitfalls of the stream the hurricane lamp came in very useful for reading the small squares of newspaper that hung from the wall on a piece of string. Up to the time I left home these squares were the only bits of serious reading I ever did. Apart from my school books of course, and quick snatches of *Peg's Paper*.

In the house we relied on oil and candles for any illumination we might need and on coal for our cooking and heating. We were never short of coal. My mother was a miner's daughter and lived in fear that one day, through strikes or some other pestilence, we would wake up and find ourselves without any. Consequently, great heaps of it lay about everywhere; under the hedges, beneath the apple tree in the front garden and blocking up the entrance to the pigsty, and in the washhouse and the barn. We had no coal-house; it had fallen to pieces long before the lavatory door fell off.

The abundance of coal was only partly due to panic buying in the summer when prices were lower. In recognition of my friendly waving from the lavatory seat, the train drivers hurled massive black boulders at me which landed almost at my feet and added considerably to the stockpile. It was usually very good quality and burned the Friday baking even blacker, and made us sweat at night.

We were less fortunate with our oil supplies. The oilman only came down when he felt like it and when all the conditions were in his favour, and even then the quantity he brought was limited to the size of his cart and the willingness of his horse. His area was farflung.

Being well acquainted with these little difficulties my mother was sparing with the lights and only lit the lamp when we could no longer see a hand in front of our face. Until then we groped about in firelight. This economy put me off the twilight hours for ever. The moment the first shadowy finger of dusk settles in a corner I rush about turning on every available light. My electric bills are enormous. I am the one all the energy-saving comments are aimed at. I am also the one who gets all the final demand letters.

If the gloaming holds no romance for me, neither do I care much for the autumn, however full of mists and mellow fruitfulness it might be for some. It was on a night in late autumn that my mother began her onslaught of the hospitals. After supper, when she had fed the pigs, boiled the potato peelings and other little delicacies for their supper the next day, battened down the fowls for the night, drawn a bucket of water from the well to see us through till morning and put enough coal on the fire to stoke a small furnace, she settled herself at the table to write her letters. This was not the simple task it would appear to be.

Above the table there was a lamp suspended by a brass chain from a beam in the ceiling. A sudden gust of wind down the chimney or a door slammed in anger was all that it took to set the lamp swinging from side to side, or round and round if the turbulence was violent enough. When this happened the variability of light and shadow that resulted made anything of a close nature such as reading, sewing, and writing letters, full of irritating interruptions. Everything hung fire until the lamp stopped swinging and normal vision was resumed. Even then the writing area of the table lay in deep shadow, causing blots and smudges to appear unexpectedly on the carefully ruled out writing paper.

Though my mother was often driven to seek my help with the spelling of the less familiar words, the style of her letters was all her own. I can never remember being asked how to spell the word 'truly' so can only assume she spelt it as she spelt it in all other formal letters that she wrote. These invariably concluded with her earnest desire to remain 'Yours Trully'. Letters to closer acquaintances and to me when eventually I left home ended with her begging us to 'Keep Smilling', which never failed to make me 'smill'.

As well as bombarding every hospital she had heard of (and many that she hadn't), with lyrical accounts of my virtues and scholastic achievements, my mother touted for references from anybody and everybody whose name was of any consequence in the outlying district. Most of them had never set eyes on me. When her importunings were successful and they replied, enclosing their opinions of me in separate sealed envelopes, she steamed open the envelopes and read the enclosures. If there was a word or a phrase that she didn't much care for she carefully scratched it out and put in something she thought would do me more justice, or she left the space open, probably thinking that what they didn't know wouldn't hurt them – or me. When it was all done to her satisfaction she sealed up the envelopes again, making frequent use of the strips of sticky paper that came round the edges of postage stamps. The finished job never quite matched up to its pristine appearance, but that was a small price to pay for the value of the adjustments she had made and their possible swinging of the polls in my favour, and it made the envelopes look more interesting.

After the letters had been written and firmly stuck down with more sticky paper it was my job to go and post them. In order to do this I had to trail up three miles of steeply winding hill before I reached the post office. The hill stood as a permanent memorial to the day I lost my faith.

When I was seven I went through a period of agonizing religious fervour which had started when God, with the help of one of my aunts, mended a bit of broken hat elastic before my mother even knew it was broken. My mother wasn't fond of sewing. The very thought of sewing, she said, was enough to make her want to fall out with her own shadow. It was in my interest to see that she had as little sewing as possible to do. When the piece of hat elastic snapped between my fingers while I was taking it off for the last time one Sunday evening after church I prayed almost without ceasing until the next Sunday that a miracle would happen and the elastic be made whole. In the best tradition of hymns ancient and modern, God worked in a mysterious way his wonders to perform. A few minutes before my mother was due to take the hat from its tissue paper and discover all, my aunt turned up unexpectedly. She got the hat out, noticed its plight, sewed the elastic back on and sent me happily to Sunday school. It is doubtful whether she ever knew that she had been chosen to be the handmaid of the Lord but I knew, and my faith was made as whole as the elastic until the fiasco of the hill destroyed it almost for ever.

I had prayed as earnestly for the hill to be removed as I had prayed for the hat elastic to be mended, but with less success. It continued to stand there, forming a weary barrier between my home and the village. However good faith might have been at moving mountains it had little effect on hills.

Chapter Three

THE ANSWERS TO the letters were slow at coming in. 'It's not a bit of use worrying about it,' said my mother when I worried. 'With Christmas nearly on top of them the hospitals will have more to do than sit about writing letters to the likes of us.' She could have been right of course. On the other hand the postman may have been to blame for some of the delay.

If writing letters was something of a hardship where we lived, getting them delivered was no easy matter either. Like the oilman, the postman only came down the lane when the weather, his state of health and his current work load permitted, he being the blacksmith, the undertaker and the wheelwright as well. Delivering letters was the most exposed of his occupations and came well down in his priorities. Postcards with such trivialities as 'Wish you were here' scrawled across them were deciphered and laid aside on his bench with circulars and other unimportant communications until he got round to dealing with them. Telegrams had to be a matter of life and death before he would consent to abandoning a coffin lid in their favour.

Errors of identification between buff-coloured envelopes containing trivia, and buff-coloured envelopes containing things of vital importance often only came to light when an irate tradesman started dunning for his money or the sugar-beet factory was late with the cheque.

Our letters were never brought to the door; the postman flatly refused to bike up the cart-track, and a wooden box had to be nailed to a tree out in the lane for him to drop them into. The paper boy availed himself of the box as did children delivering messages from their mother to mine. It was one of my first jobs in the morning to get at the box before marauding wildlife made confetti of the contents.

Since there was nothing that could be done about getting me off to be a nurse until the replies started coming in my mother went on with the preparations for Christmas as usual. These included making arrangements for the pig-killing.

On the day booked well in advance – he was much in demand – the butcher arrived with an assortment of well-honed knives and a length of rope. As in home midwifery my mother rushed about keeping him plenteously supplied with kettles of boiling water. I stayed in the house and kept my ears covered to protect them from the raucous squeals of the stuck pig. Living so close to us by the kitchen door, if it had been with us for a long time and I had become attached to it, the noise it made could be very upsetting for me.

For the next few days our house was full of the smell of baking and boiling, of sage and onions, thyme and parsley and fat joints of pork sizzling and crackling in the oven. Steam ran down the windows obliterating the outside world and the noise of grinding and chopping drowned all other noises.

When the fever was over, the beams in our kitchen were festooned with trailing links of glistening sausages, every dish in the house was taken up with something delicious, and on the living-room walls, between the pictures of 'Betrothed' and 'Wedded', and my uncle Jack who lost an arm in the Great War, hung the huge sides of bacon and the hams that my father had cured in the barn with lumps of saltpetre. And I came out in spots and no wonder at it. I also got fat which was not surprising either.

Meals in our house were never balanced. My mother knew nothing about balancing meals. She cooked what she knew we liked and plenty of it, and got cross if we left any. Cholesterol, like Judgement Day, was something to be reckoned with later. And when it was too late to do anything much about it.

Because of the poor dead pig hanging from the walls

our diet owed much of its bulk to bacon. For breakfast we ate several slices of boiled streaky with hard boiled eggs on the side. My father swilled the meal down with pints of black sweet tea, but I had to drink milky cocoa which often collided with the fatty bacon inside me. My mother was a great believer in milky cocoa for growing children, whichever way it made them grow. She was an authority on what was good for growing children. Once, on the farm where we used to live, she had threatened to report the waggoner's wife to the cruelty inspector for giving her children cereal and coffee for breakfast instead of boiled bacon and cocoa. My mother didn't believe in cereals. She didn't believe in coffee either. There was something a little sinful about both commodities.

Dinner was a hearty midday meal of savoury suet pudding or Yorkshire pudding served as a sort of hors d'oeuvre before the main course, followed by a stack of vegetables and meat, and for afters something like a jam roly-poly or a spotted dick. Whichever it happened to be, we ate it liberally coated with rice pudding or rich egg custard, plus an extra layer of hot jam or marmalade.

For supper, to make a change from bacon, we had boiled ham accompanied by great slabs of thickly buttered bread, two sorts of cake and Bakewell tart or a piece of apple pie to round off the meal. This left ample space for bread and cheese and cocoa before we went to bed.

To combat the spots that covered my chin my mother gave me massive doses of brimstone and treacle every Saturday night after I had had my bath.

On Saturday night a tin bath was brought in from the wash-house, a couple of kettles of boiling water were thrown into it, the temperature brought down to a degree or two above freezing point and we dipped ourselves in and out of it as fast as we could. Like going round the back, bathing was something we did from necessity. It was never a luxury to be lingered over. In spite of the fire that expended its energies halfway up the living-room chimney, our kitchen was a very draughty place; the wind whistled through the back door and the window frames.

The reason Saturday night was chosen for our ablutions was so that we and our underwear would be without stain for the Sabbath. This weekly purification may not have been so necessary for my father, who in my memory had never set foot inside a church, but for my mother and me, who both sang in the choir, it was important that we at least set out clean. Whether we stayed clean or not during the three-mile journey depended to a large extent on whether we got a puncture somewhere along the way. Getting a puncture could ruin a good bath. It could ruin a lot of other things as well, including tempers.

Not only did my mother sing in the choir but she cleaned the church, polished its brasses, did its flowers, washed its surplices and made its vicar's life a misery. He was terrified of her. She bent him to her will whenever a decision had to be made, whether it concerned the hymns we were to sing on Sunday or where we should go on the choir outing. We always went to Skegness; my mother couldn't abide Mablethorpe or Cleethorpes.

The gentle vicar must have spent many weary hours in his study every week vetting his sermon and the hymns for words that could jeopardize their message. My mother didn't approve of words like 'bosom' so whenever we sang 'Jesu lover of my soul' she stopped singing immediately before the anatomical detail in the second line was due to crop up and resumed in full voice once the gathering waters were reached. The abrupt cessation of her powerful contralto voice brought the choir boys into direct confrontation with their bosom fantasies and the singing became very erratic until she restored order by whacking one or two of the offenders over the head with her hymn book. 'Bowels' caused the same happy confusion. The vicar had to choose his Old Testament readings with extra care.

It was during choir practice that I first heard about sex. Brian Taylor gave me the details during a short interval between two psalms. He seemed well up in his subject and with one or two reservations about the vicar and my parents I believed every word he told me, but not for long.

Every week a small magazine called *Peg's Paper* was dropped in the box down the lane. It was only after Brian had drawn aside the fig leaf enough to give me a fascinating glimpse of what lay beneath that the covers of the magazines started to interest me. The pictures on them were invariably of a young woman and a tall dark and handsome young man clutching each other from a distance of about six inches. What they were saying could only be guessed at from the agonized – passionate – rapturous or just plain stupid look on their faces. Until Brian's startling revelations about the behaviour of adults I had never given the covers a second glance, dismissing them as soppy. But after that, it all took on a new significance for me. When I had fetched up the magazines with the *Nottingham Journal* and anything else that might have been in the box, my mother grabbed them off me and stuffed them under the cushion of her rocking chair, presumably so that my already tarnished innocence should not be corrupted further by their contents. Alas for her good intentions, I had usually read enough coming up the cart-track to whet my appetite for more. Whenever I got the chance I tucked one of them up my knicker leg and went round the back to have a quick read; either by the light of the sun or the hurricane lamp. It was when I came to the bit where the young lady, blushing rosily, was astounding her equally naive young husband with the news that a little stranger was shortly to bless their union that it occurred to me that Brian had been having me on. When I tackled him about it later he had to admit that he also had been misinformed. For why – we asked ourselves, if the husband had done all he was supposed to have done to implant the little stranger – would he need to be warned of its impending arrival?

It was a long time before all the mysteries were unravelled for me. The few details that Brian had given me, which turned out to be surprisingly accurate, plus the bits I picked up at the back of the school bus and in the hockey shed on wet days, were all the sex education I ever got. If our mothers knew anything about such things in those days they kept it to themselves and the facts of life our teachers taught us were not nearly as interesting.

Not only did we bike to church twice on Sundays, and in the afternoon as well if there was anything worth going for, but my mother and I never missed any of the entertainments it laid on for our pleasure. These included harvest suppers, christenings, funerals, weddings and the annual village social. This was the highlight of our lives.

As well as playing games, each of us was expected to oblige with a party piece. None of us needed any encouragement to comply with this condition of entry; we would have been bitterly disappointed if we had not been asked. I recited 'The Way through the Woods' which never aroused much interest, and my mother sang 'Let the Rest of the World Go By' which did. Years later when the song got back in the charts I astonished my teenage daughters at the speed I picked up the words. I didn't like to tell them how long it had been around and how good their grandmother was at singing it.

It was while we were playing musical chairs one evening that the baker's daughter ran screaming into the Victory Hall to tell us that the mail train had fallen over in a nearby field. We hurried down the dark lane to where the great engine lay on its side in a ditch with pitiful indignity. The older children among us were given the responsibility of standing on the running boards of cars belonging to the gentry, holding down quickly improvised stretchers on their way to the hospital. Others simply knelt on the railway bank and held people's hands. There were many dresses, *crêpe de Chine* and other more sophisticated ones, that would never be worn again when that night was over.

For me the accident was a foretaste of things to come. If only I had been a born nurse I might have learnt a lot of valuable lessons from it. As it was, all it did for me was give me nightmares for a long time after, which surely should have told somebody something. It didn't, and the plans for turning me into a nurse went on regardless.

Chapter Four

CHRISTMAS WAS OVER and the last of the plum puddings had been wrapped in a clean cloth and stored away for Easter Sunday before the official-looking letters started to be dropped in the box. When they did and we studied them it was soon obvious even to us that the voluntary hospitals had not been impressed by my mother's account of my virtues and scholastic achievements; neither had the repair jobs with the sticky paper nor the amendments to the testimonials done anything to influence them in my favour. In every case they had expected more than I was able to offer them. Their letters were polite but chilly; they all added up to the same thing – they didn't want me. Their rejection of me upset my mother very much. She boiled up more at every one she read. 'It just goes to show,' she grumbled furiously, 'you never can tell about some things. And after all the sacrifices we made to send you to the high school and the nice things I put about you in the vicar's letter you'd have thought they'd have jumped at you.'

She would have stormed even louder and certainly a lot longer if the salary they were offering had sounded more promising. As it was, it started at twelve pounds a year and rose in barely perceptible annual increments to reach a less than staggering climax of twenty pounds at the end of three years. Even I, unversed as I was in high finance, saw nothing enticing about it. I was later to learn that the honour of becoming a voluntary-trained nurse was supposed to be sufficient recompense in itself without the added bait of inflated salaries. This propaganda put about by voluntary-trained nurses made them snobby with the rest of the profession for a long time.

Their proud boast was a left-over from the days when nurses worked for love or gin – never both. It was only after the Second World War, when a new Health Act paved the way for revolution in the hospital service, that the two started to merge, and even then it was a long time before people came round to believing that nurses could work for love and still enjoy a little gin on the side, or at least enough money to pay for the gin if their taste ran in that direction. Miss Nightingale undoubtedly did wonders for nursing but not so much for nurses. When she went, she left behind her an image of a winged and haloed angel who could never be tempted by anything as filthy as lucre. Nurses are still fighting to live down that image.

The letters from the municipal hospitals were much kinder to me. They were more tolerant with my short-comings, and being state-aided could afford to be more generous with their money. They lured my mother on with dazzling offers of eighteen pounds a year to start with, rising to twenty-five on the day I became a State Registered Nurse with all its accompanying responsibilities.

'That sounds a lot better,' she said. 'What with your food and washing thrown in as well.' She read and re-read the letters looking for hidden snags and it was to a municipal hospital that she finally presented me for inspection.

Throughout the interview I never once opened my mouth. I didn't have to. My mother said all there was to be said. She answered questions and made promises in my name like a good conscientious godparent, occasionally glancing across at me as if expecting some support but never waiting long enough to get any.

I listened to what she was saying with acute embarrassment. By no stretch of the imagination could I have fitted the identikit she was drawing of me. One look at me was enough to tell anybody that I was not the unselfish girl, devoted to animals, children, the elderly and the sick that she was making me out to be. Nevertheless the Matron must have believed some of it for we left the hospital with a drawn-up contract to start my training on my eighteenth birthday and a list an arm long of things I would need to have before I started.

The list gave us a lot of trouble. There were things on it we had never heard of, or had only read about in advertisements in the Sunday papers. One of these was a dressing gown. There had never been such a thing in our house. We knew all there was to know about winceyette nightdresses, but nothing about dressing gowns. Having no bathroom to pop in and out of a dressing gown would have been quite superfluous. Neither had we ever needed a dressing gown for sitting about being ill in. Nobody was ever ill in our house. My mother didn't believe in illness. She believed that if you were firm enough with it or ignored it completely, like a naughty child it would get better, which it did.

Perhaps one of the reasons why we were never ill was because we had our own remedies for arresting small complaints before they got any bigger. Things like brimstone for my spots and the family bowels, plenty of cold water from the well to drink if we felt a cold coming on, and butter and sugar worked together with a drop or two of vinegar to stop a mild cough becoming a nasty hacking one. All the remedies worked. Or if they didn't we had to suffer – in silence – until the ailment got better of its own accord.

For more serious complaints, like fingers almost severed in turnip cutters, or bone-deep gashes with scythes, there was always a slice of mouldy cheese in the damp larder for my father to slap on the wound and tie down firmly with a clean red spotted handkerchief. We didn't call it penicillin but it worked the same, even if it took longer.

After we had studied the list the hospital had given us and pondered over its mysteries my mother put on her hat and coat and got our bikes out of the barn.

'We'd better ride up to the village and let Sam have a look at this,' she said. Sam was the proprietor of our local shop. We trusted in him to put us right on certain things. Our trust was sadly misplaced. He pored over the list for a long time then had to admit there was little he could do for us. He knew almost as little about dressing gowns as we did and absolutely nothing about other small items that were mentioned.

'I've got a watch or two,' he said, producing a cardboard box from under the counter, 'but they all seem to be men's.' He was right. They were all very large and made to be threaded on a chain and slung across the abdomen. In spite of the fact that they had the second hand the list had made such a point of mentioning, I clearly needed a watch that encircled my wrist.

The bust bodices he showed us were just as useless. They were made of pink brioche, rigidly boned and fashioned for ladies more amply endowed than I was in that area. Sam did his best, he was determined not to lose a customer.

'I shouldn't worry about them being a bit on the big side,' he said helpfully. 'They're bound to shrink a couple of inches when you wash them, but if its the colour you don't like, well I know for a fact they fade to white if you give them a good boiling in the copper.' We believed him but my mother refused to take the risk of them emerging from the suds as large and pink as when they went in. She looked doubtfully round the shop.

'I think we'll go to the Co-op and see what they've got,' she said at last. Sam looked very put out but she stood her ground, and after her abortive attempt at local patronage we went to the Co-op to do our shopping.

Whatever else my mother did not believe in, and there was plenty, she was a firm believer in the Co-op. She was also a firm believer in the Tory party, which indicated that somewhere along the line the aims and ideals of the Labour party for the brotherhood of man had escaped her.

It was during our orgy of shopping at the Co-op that I fought, and won, the only battle I ever remember having with my mother. It was over a pair of combinations. I had worn 'coms' ever since I left off wearing Liberty bodices, and I hated them. They were extremely ugly garments that encased the body from neck to knees, leaving suitable apertures for natural functions. Over each bosom a double layer of material was inserted. This was intended to be removed by nursing mothers during periods of lactation. I was determined to start my new life without the indignity of coms. The emancipated shop-girl who was serving us joined in the battle and between us we defeated my mother.

'Nobody wears them things these days,' said the girl with an air of authority. My mother took no notice of her and went on fingering the goods to assess their quality. Unfortunately they were made in England and of the finest.

'Nobody wears them these days,' I chimed in nervously. My mother took no notice of me either. She picked up the coms and examined them from all angles.

'I left off wearing them a long time ago,' persisted the girl, now realizing what was at stake. My mother flushed angrily.

'What you do or what you don't wear is no concern of mine, young lady. If your mother hasn't any more sense than to let you go round without coms that's her look out.' And that seemed to be final, but the girl wasn't so easily put off.

'They've gone up you know,' she said, hiding the price tag under the counter. 'They're three and eleven now, not three and six like they was last week, that's fivepence three farthings more a pair.' My mother looked at her suspiciously. The girl dropped the price tag out of sight.

My mother did a bit of quick arithmetic in her head and weighed up the advantages of winning the battle against the inflated cost of three pairs of combinations. Thrift won.

As well as leading me into victorious battle against my mother the same emancipated shop-girl introduced us to the small items that Sam up in the village had confessed to having no knowledge of at all. These were small cotton wool contrivances that had apparently been invented to replace the squares of old bits of sheet material that had to be boiled for long hours in the copper every month to restore them to their original whiteness. We listened to the girl's account of their usefulness in silence. She was very informative.

'All you have to do when they're finished with is wrap them up in a bit of newspaper and throw them in the fire,' she told us without batting an eyelid. My mother refused to meet my eye. Such personal things had never been mentioned before.

After we had bought several packets of the useful but unmentionable articles and finished the rest of our shopping we trailed back up the cart-track with our parcels. In them were: six pairs of fleecy-lined navy-blue knickers, bought to offset the shock to my system of being deprived of combinations; enough black woollen stockings to last a year with careful darning, which they never got though they still had to last a year; two pairs of comfortable house shoes that would be worn out long before they provided any comfort to my aching feet; watch with second hand, fountain pen, propelling pencil and a dressing gown in a brilliant Highland plaid that no Highlander would have been seen dead in despite the Co-op's assurances that they were all the rage.

On top of this formidable expenditure my mother had been instructed by the hospital to write to a firm in Manchester that specialized in nurses' uniform, enclosing my vital statistics, an order for several sets of uniform and a postal order to cover the cost. Also to a firm of publishers for books on anatomy, physiology and hygiene, and a nurses' dictionary which, after more than forty years, I still have.

When the books arrived from the publishers one look at them was enough to send my mother off in a rush to stuff them under the cushion with the current edition of *Peg's Paper*. That the whole point of turning me into a nurse was so that I would familiarize myself with their contents in the shortest possible time made no difference to her. She would have died sooner than let me get a glimpse of some of the colour plates while I was still a child under her roof.

As the days flew past the butterflies in my stomach fluttered about in nervous panic at the thought of my impending departure, my father called me 'Birdie' more often and my mother started making small overtures of affection that were as embarrassing to her as they were for me.

The butterflies' behaviour was predictable but the other two phenomena were not. My father was a quiet man who never spoke two words where one would do. Neither did he ever call my mother or me by our first names. If he had ever known my mother's first name he had forgotten it long ago, she was always 'Missis' to him. On the rare occasions that he needed a name for me he called me 'Birdie', which made me feel warm and comfortable inside. It probably originated from the days when I took his snap down to the fields and he fed me from the point of his clasp knife as well as the birds. That he was using the name more often was an indication that he was suffering a little at the thought of me leaving the nest. It was the only indication he ever showed.

We were all vastly relieved when my mother stopped trying to be affectionate and went back to being her usual brisk no-nonsense self. But before she did she seized the opportunity to have a little talk to me.

'Mind you behave yourself when you go away. I don't want you getting yourself into no trouble if you know what I mean.' I knew what she meant and we carefully avoided each other for the rest of the day.

A day or two before I was due to leave home we went upstairs and moved the apples that were always stored beneath my bed. We dragged out the large tin trunk that had lain there with the apples for many years, emptied it and threw away the brass-bound books that nobody had ever read. Their mustiness conveyed itself to my clothes and for a long time I went about smelling like a disused library.

When we started packing my things I noticed that my mother was folding them in such a way that it was impossible for me to read the name tapes she had sewn on them after I went to bed at night. There was something about this obvious secrecy that bothered me. I was soon to know the reason for it.

Chapter Five

IF BRINGING ME up, educating me and choosing a career for me had given my mother a minimum of headaches, imparting the news that she wasn't really my mother at all gave her no more pain – at least on the surface. She remained calm throughout the disclosures and left the hysterics to me. Mine didn't last long either, though I thoroughly enjoyed them while they lasted.

The day before I left home she called me into the living-room. Her voice had none of its usual sharpness and when I went in to her she was sitting on the edge of her rocking chair looking a bit uncomfortable. The thought of what she might be going to say to me made me feel just as uncomfortable. All I could think it might be was an enlargement on the theme of what would happen to me if I didn't behave myself when I left home. I couldn't have been more wrong.

I stood in front of her and we looked everywhere but at each other for a long time. At last she spoke.

'You'd better sit down,' she said. 'There's something I've got to tell you.' I sat down and immediately stood up again. We went on looking at each other until, seized by a sudden attack of nervous incontinence, I excused myself and escaped round the back. I sat among the winter-stricken nettles for as long as I dared, hoping that by the time I got back into the house things would have returned to normal. They hadn't. My mother abruptly came to the point.

'You don't belong to us,' she said in a loud, defensive voice. I stared at her in horror, wondering what I could have possibly done to make her so anxious to disown me after all those years. With all my faults I could think of none that merited such total rejection. She went on talking.

'We took you in when you were a baby. Your father was killed in the war you see and your mother couldn't afford to keep you. They wasn't married.'

I sat stunned and speechless, turning over in my mind the things she had told me, which amounted to very little. I dwelt for a moment on a harrowing picture of my natural father, young and handsome, and bleeding to death on some foreign battlefield then I burst into tears. The mother who had taken me in when I was a baby ignored my tears.

'We never adopted you properly so your real name's different from ours. Your first name's different as well,

I called you after a girl I used to go to school with.' I perked up a bit at this. I had never been fond of any of my names and the thought of getting a whole new set looked like making up for some of the shocks I had had that afternoon.

Leaving my father to his fate on the battlefield I turned my thoughts to my poor young mother. I pictured her shawled and bonneted, with me in her arms, being turned out into the cold snow by an irate father, with nowhere to go and not a penny to bless herself with, and my tears flowed anew. I sat egging myself on to fresh paroxysms of grief until my less romantic mother got up from her rocking chair and went upstairs. I heard the floorboards in her bedroom creaking and the sound of drawers being opened and shut. When she came down again she was carrying a tin box. My mother took the lid off and a few petals from some old pressed flowers fell to the floor. They lay on the pegged rag rug looking small and lost. She turned over a collection of faded photographs, some glossy greetings cards and a lot of black-edged letters.

'Here,' she said, handing me an official-looking document. 'You'd better have a look at this. It's your birth certificate, you'll need it for exams and things. The Matron knows all about it and she said you were to start using your proper name when you got there. You'd better start learning it so you'll know it off by heart.' I took the paper from her and had a good look at it. My heart sank. I could see at a glance that I was going to have trouble with my surname. It was a new one to me and would take some remembering. I made a spot decision to abandon the first of the first names in favour of the second. Florence was as bad as the one I already had and apart from which it seemed presumptuous to suddenly assume the name of the Lady of the Lamp before I had even set foot inside a hospital.

But the thing that had me staring at the document with open mouth was that I was born in London. I was a Londoner, perhaps even a cockney, most certainly a foreigner. It was the most amazing thing to come out of that afternoon: that I, who had lived all my life in Lincolnshire, should turn out to be a Londoner. When all the other discoveries had become commonplace through use, that was to remain a constant amazement.

Without another word my mother wrote down my name on a bit of paper and put the birth certificate in an envelope ready for me to take to the hospital with me. From that day the matter was never once mentioned again.

My mother had ordered the carrier's cart to be at the house prompt at two on the Saturday I was to leave, which gave her, me, and my trunk ample time to catch the three o'clock train to Nottingham. All morning none of us said much; there was nothing left for us to say. My father avoided my eye. He had evidently been told that I knew he was not my father and this placed him in a very peculiar position.

My mother and I packed the few things that had been left out till the last minute then wandered about until dinner-time getting on each other's nerves.

When dinner-time came my appetite had gone. This surprised me very much. It took a lot to put me off my food. The day I had my tonsils out I came straight home and ate the dinner my mother had kept hot for me. But today was different. Today my stomach was in no state to welcome food.

When the carrier arrived he heaved my mother and the trunk on the back of his cart while I lingered behind and plucked up enough courage to kiss my father for what may have been the first time in my life. Kissing had never been encouraged much in our house. My mother didn't believe in it. Nevertheless my father seemed to enjoy it though he took no active part in the proceedings. As I picked my way through the bristles – he only shaved on Wednesdays and Sundays so Saturday was not a good day to inaugurate the custom – I thought of the little picnics in the fields when I took his snap down to him, and the squeak of his leather leggings as he walked with me down the lanes, and my sudden tears forged a love that would never be usurped by an unknown father, however nobly he may have died for his King and country.

When I had finished kissing him and before he lifted me on to the cart with my mother, my father dug into the pocket of his stained old corduroy trousers and brought out a little leather bag tied up with string.

From the bag he took four green and scarcely recognizable half-crowns and gave them to me. 'Be a good girl, Birdie,' he said and turned away quickly. I accepted the windfall gratefully; it was more than I had ever had to call my own and the jingling of the coins temporarily dried my tears.

We arrived at the hospital at six as we had been warned to do and were shown into a waiting room by a girl whose greeting was less than friendly.

'So you've come at last,' she said, very huffily. 'It's about time too, I shudder been off at five. It's always the same in this place. Them as will may. Give us your trunk.' We apologized humbly for being prompt and she staggered away with my trunk balanced precariously in her thin arms. Her progress down the corridor was marked by dull thuds and piercing screams but after a while the sounds died down and there was silence.

We sat stiffly on two of the chairs that lined the walls. As the time passed my mother began to get very fidgety and started looking at the clock and at me. She wasn't used to being away from home at such a late hour. At last she could bear it no longer. She stood up and fastened her coat which she had undone so that she would feel the benefit when she got out, picked her umbrella off the floor, opened her handbag to make sure she had the return ticket safe and looked at me.

'Now remember what I told you about behaving yourself,' she said. 'I'd better be getting back before your father starts worrying.' She gave me a quick peck on the cheek, pressed another half-a-crown in my hand and went. I was glad to see her go. It was a moment I had been dreading, but now that it was over I realized there was nothing to be gained by her staying. Already she, my father, and the little house up the cart-track were being lost sight of in the excitement of new beginnings.

Chapter Six

I SAT FOr a long time after my mother had left. Occasionally someone walked in and looked at me. Then, not liking or not wanting what they saw, they went away again without speaking. I began to feel cold and hungry and a bit desolate. I began to wish I had never come to be a nurse since nobody seemed to want me. I wished there was a table in front of me laden with ham and eggs, currant cake and jam pasties. I wished I was anywhere but where I was, waiting for I knew not what.

At last a woman peered in at the door. She was very large, and very terrifying. She had on a blue and white outfit that crackled when she moved. It was topped by a lacy bonnet that had been worked on lovingly and for a long time with a goffering iron, the sort my mother did the frills on the choir boys' surplices with. It made each frill stand out separately, independent of its neighbour.

Seeing me sitting there the woman rushed in, grabbed me by the arm and pulled me off the chair. 'Good gracious, child, what on earth are you sitting here for?'

she shrieked. 'You must be the new nurse. Why hasn't somebody taken you to your room? You should be upstairs getting ready for supper. You'd better come with me.' I went with her, my knees shaking. Being called a nurse, albeit a new one, had robbed me of all speech but my escort seemed to expect none from me and she rushed on ahead, with me careering after her.

We tore down corridors and up stairs. Everywhere was done out in the same dull shades of brown and green and everywhere was badly in need of re-doing. The gloom of the colour scheme did nothing to relieve my gloom and I was glad when we pulled up sharp outside a door.

The room we went into was small and dark. I looked at the walls in despair. They were as dingy as the corridors had been. I was used to seeing wallpaper in bedrooms, with lovebirds hanging from boughs of apple trees and bright floral sprays in between. In one of our bedrooms at home there had been a paper which from a distance appeared to be dotted with rows of fried eggs tastefully arranged on willow-pattern dinner plates. It was only when you moved in closer that the eggs became yellow roses and the dinner plates turned out to be lace doilies. At least it gave you something to look at when you woke up in the morning, which was more than could be said for the distemper I was to live with for the next few years.

Jostling each other in the tiny room were three dressing tables, one prehistoric wardrobe and three iron beds. There was a precision about the way the beds were made that had me worried from the start. I knew it was something I would never be able to compete with. In spite of my mother's careful training, I was not of a neat and tidy disposition, which was something that had caused a considerable amount of friction between us. The woman was not impressed by the neatness of the beds. She took one look at the two that were presumably not to be mine, muttered something that I didn't quite catch, then rushed across to them and started tearing the bedding off them. She did it with such fury that I shrank back, expecting every minute for her to seize a hairbrush from one of the dressing tables and whack me over the head with it. She didn't and I stopped trembling. When the last sheet had been stripped off and the last pillow lay on the floor she came back to me. She was panting heavily and her hair had shed a few pins and was sticking out of her cap in several places.

'These beds are a disgrace,' she breathed. 'I hope I never find yours looking like that.' She looked at me accusingly, and I felt she was holding me responsible in some way for the two beds. She hoped in vain. There was hardly a night that I didn't come off duty, worn out and longing for my bed, only to find it stripped to the springs. For the first week or two it was as much as I could do to drag the mattress into place – if she had torn that off as well in her fury – and fall across it, still with my clothes on and asleep before the hardness of the flock-filled thing I was lying on began to seep through to my body. It was a long time before I was able to muster enough energy to reassemble the blankets and sheets in their proper order before stumbling wearily between them.

The woman helped me to unpack my trunk. Between us we laid the Co-op lingerie, negligee, and other sundries in an orderly crush in two narrow drawers of the dressing table that had been allotted to me, and hung the hangables in my section of the wardrobe which, like my father's old armchair, was suffering from an attack of woodworm still in its active stage. The smell of moth balls and must that escaped when the door was opened was the perfect foil for the old-book smell of my clothing.

While we worked she talked. She told me that she was the home-sister, laying great stress on the importance of the position. She explained that she was responsible for seeing that the nurses behaved themselves while they were in the home and kept the rules that were made to be kept – not broken.

'Never let me find your bed not made or your drawers untidy,' she said, looking at me as angrily as if she had already discovered both.

'No, Miss,' I promised.

'And don't call me Miss, kindly remember to call me Sister.'

'Yes, Miss,' I said obediently. She drew in a sharp breath and turned purple. 'Yes, Sister,' I amended.

'And don't let me find you sitting about in your room or smoking in it,' she said, mollified by my correction. 'There is a sitting-room for you to sit in and a library for you to smoke in, though why any decent girl should wish to smoke I cannot think.'

I seized the opportunity to get myself into her good books. 'Please, Miss, I don't smoke,' I said, glad of the word in edgeways. I was wasting my breath. She turned on me furiously.

'Whether you smoke or not is beside the point, the point I am trying to make is that I never want to find you smoking in your room.'

'No, Miss,' I said, submissively. She drew in another sharp breath but let my slip pass.

'And never let me see you leave the nurses' home looking untidy, or coming into it late. Ten o'clock is the time for you to be in if you have an evening off, though what a young lady wants to be out as late as ten o'clock at night for I simply do not know.' Neither did I, never having been out as late as ten o'clock at night, but having learned my lesson with the bit about not smoking I kept quiet. She went on.

'If I find you doing any of the things I have told you not to do, or not doing the things I have told you to do, I shall give you warning myself the first time but after that you will be sent to the Matron for her to deal with you.' As my mother was kind enough to observe about girls who had babies before they were married, you could forgive the first but not the second.

What the home-sister had not told me and what I was soon to learn for myself was that she combined the duties of home-sister with the vigilance of a prison wardress. A kind wardress sometimes but a wardress nevertheless.

Her name was Mary. She had a surname of course but it was never used except to her face. Behind her back she was always Mary – Bloody Mary if she had been more than usually vindictive. She was guardian angel and avenging angel set in authority over all lesser angels. The angelic host she ruled over loved or hated her according to the number of times she stripped their beds or tipped their untidy drawers on to the floor, or caught them not only sitting but smoking in their rooms, or accosted them going out or coming in improperly dressed or at the wrong time or by the wrong route. Nothing escaped her eagle eye. Nobody set foot inside or outside the home without a quick look round to see whether she was about. Usually she was, waiting in a corner or behind a door ready to pounce and hold for questioning until her questions had been answered to her satisfaction. A nurse going innocently to her room could expect to be waylaid.

'Where are you going, Nurse?'

'To my room, Sister.'

'And what for, may I ask?'

'Please, Sister, to change my apron.'

'Then be quick about it and don't let me come in and find you sitting on your bed.'

'No, Sister. Thank you, Sister.' If the nurse happened to be travelling towards the front door instead of away from it the interrogation took a different line.

'And where do you think you are going, Nurse?'

'Please, Sister, out.'

If it was later than six in the evening the next question was inevitable.

'And have you got a pass, Nurse?'

'No, Sister.'

'Then see that you are in not a minute later than ten.'

'Yes, Sister. Thank you, Sister.' The gratitude was presumably in recognition of not getting a beating.

When my trunk had finally been emptied and my clothes arranged in the way the home-sister would expect to find them for the next three years and longer she sorted out a set of uniform for me to put on in the morning. She put in studs and rubber buttons and explained where everything had to go and why. It was all very complicated, especially the cap. She got very irritable over the cap. Not only was I untidy by nature but I was also clumsy with my fingers. It took me a long time to grasp all she was trying to tell me about how to make a cap. Having to convert a large square of material into a small and wearable butterfly cap gave me a lot of trouble. The caps I made were either too big or too small, and slipped over one eye or slid off the back of my head; they were never where they should have been. I realized afterwards that this was the sort of thing that never happened to born nurses. Their caps were invariably masterpieces of architectural symmetry and neither slipped nor slid. The angle she wore her cap was the hallmark of a born nurse.

After the set of uniform and the cap had been laid across a chair ready for the morning, the sister took me down to supper. For a reason that nobody could ever explain, the dining-room in my training school was called the mess-room. The name was an unfortunate choice, for not only did it make the place seem drearier than it already was, but it provided a launching pad for a lot of poor jokes about the quality of the food that was served there. However poor the jokes were the food was usually even poorer.

The room was large and bleak and extremely noisy when a meal was in progress. Four bare tables stretched along its full length and a fifth stood in splendid isolation well away from the serving hatch. This was where the sisters sat. They were never put off their food by the smell of stale cabbage that drifted in from the kitchen whenever the hatch door was opened.

At the four tables sat the nurses in strict order of seniority, from the staff-nurses, who were only slightly less exalted than the sisters, down to the last of the juniors which that night, and until the next one came, was me.

As well as the more obvious segregation of the ranks by the separate tables there were several finer distinctions made at each table, the nurse at the bottom end automatically becoming the dog's body for all the other nurses. Her position improved in single stages until she reached the summit. Then the slow climb began again at the next table. Only when she reached the glittering apex of the staff-nurses' table was she entirely free from the chores that had kept her busy during the years she was a probationer. The demands made on the lower orders were so time-consuming it was a miracle they ever got anything to eat at all. Their meal-times were spent passing up cruets, passing across jugs of water, hacking off slices of bread for anyone senior to themselves if by but a day, and rushing to and from the hatch for fresh supplies. The mess-room maids concentrated on the sisters and left the nurses to do their own slaving, the more junior being the greater in bondage.

Before I left school I went with a few other girls to have my fortune told. The woman we went to was supposed to be very good at it. She had a great reputation for being able to locate lost cattle for local farmers, and was often able to help the police with their inquiries. We hadn't lost any cattle nor were we wanting help with our inquiries; we just went for the fun of it.

When it came to my turn to go into the front room where the fortune teller lay on the sofa in a state of trance, I expected to be told romantic things about the colour of my future husband's eyes and how many children I was likely to have. Instead, she grasped my hand tightly in hers and started thrashing about on the sofa saying incomprehensible things.

'You can jolly well cut your own bread tomorrow,' she hissed at me, with beads of perspiration breaking out on her brow. 'You wait until I'm a senior, I'll never cut another slice of bread for anybody as long as I live.' As cut bread had still to be invented, what she was saying made no sense at all to me. I listened to her ramblings and could only conclude that she had suddenly gone mad. When she sat up and asked for the threepence that was her fee for the session I felt I had been sadly cheated: especially when all the other girls, with one exception, had been told the things I had gone there to hear. The one exception hadn't been told anything. The woman had even refused to take her money. When the girl was knocked off her bicycle and killed by a passing motorist barely a week later, the coincidence did nothing to change my opinion of unscrupulous fortune tellers. It was only after I had spent a lot of my mealtimes sawing off bread for my seniors that I began to wonder whether there might not be something in fortune telling after all.

That night, being not yet in uniform, I was excused the duties that would be mine in the morning. I sat at the bottom of the most junior table and waited. I waited a long time before anybody noticed me and by the time they did and slapped a plate in front of me there were no potatoes left and the cabbage had all gone. The brownish substance on the plate turned out to be stew, or the hospital equivalent of stew. It had me guessing for a long time.

Stews in our house were thick, aromatic, mouth-watering regalements, the result of much loving preparation and long hours of slow cooking. They were laced with pot-herbs and dumplings. There was nothing recognizable in the watery mixture that fell persistently through the prongs of my fork. The rice pudding that followed was even more watery and reminded me of a little girl I had once heard describing the rice pudding her granny had given her for dinner.

'Granny's graby was lovely, Mummy, but her peas was ever so hard.' Even the graby wasn't lovely but being hungry I ate it all. I lost my way back to the bedroom several times.

Eminent naturalists can often be heard on the wireless going into ecstasies over the mating of two earthworms, leaving the rest of us to wonder what we have been missing all our lives. Switching on the electric light in the bedroom filled me with the same sort of ecstasy. Never had I wielded such power. The brilliance that flooded the room at my slightest touch threw me into a passion of discovery. I went on pushing the switch up and down until I was satisfied that the miracle was no flash in the pan then I sat down on the bed wondering what was going to happen next. I wasn't left wondering for long. Soon after nine o'clock the door burst open and two girls fell into the room. They were both in uniform and were both about my age. One of them was tall and thin with flaming red hair and very big feet. The reason I noticed her feet was because she had her shoes in her hand and there were gaping holes in both her stockings. The other girl was short and plump and spotty like me. She also had her shoes in her hand and gaping holes in her stockings. After a quick glance in my direction they decided to carry on as if I wasn't there. When they saw the bedding on the floor they gave wild shrieks and flew across the room. 'My God,' they roared in chorus. 'That bloody old Mary's been round again and stripped our beds. That's the second time she's done it today.' Again I got the feeling that I was being held responsible. They picked up the mattresses and hurled them back on the beds with the rest of the things, while I sat watching and listening.

'God,' groaned the red-headed one, 'my feet are killing me.' She dropped the pillow she was hammering at and clutched one of her feet in her hands. With the other she danced dangerously round the room. 'And that bloody staff-nurse has been on at me all day. I'm fed up with nursing.' My heart turned cold.

'And me,' said the other, also nursing her damaged feet. 'Never mind, it's change day tomorrow. Things might get a bit better then.'

The other refused to be comforted. 'That staff-nurse is a bitch,' she said bitterly. 'She's done nothing but make my life a misery for the past three months.' She relapsed into foot-sore silence. I was horrified at the words I had heard. I had never before heard the name of God used except in a religious context and 'bloody' was something that only rude boys at the back of the school bus said when they were showing off in front of us girls. And as for the other awful word, even my father only said lady dogs in front of me. I trembled to think what my mother would have thought if she could have heard them.

The girls went on talking loudly and importantly and obviously for my benefit about bowels and bladders, and other such indelicate things. Both of them spoke in accents that were foreign to me. I discovered later that the red-haired one was from Ireland and the other from Wales, but never having met anybody before from either country, they could have been immigrants from another hemisphere for all I knew. As well as saying 'God' a lot the red-haired one included the three members of the Holy Family into her conversation just as if they were next-door neighbours, which shocked me even more than 'God' had done. Jesus, Mary and Joseph were far too sacred to be spoken of lightly.

When they had finished making their beds they both started getting undressed. At my home, getting undressed was a very private thing, almost as private as going round the back. My mother would not have removed her blouse without hiding herself behind a door to do it and I had never in my life seen my father without so much as a sock. The two girls completely disregarded the rules of modesty. They took off each garment with no attempt at concealment. When they got as far as their bust bodices I turned my head away, but not before I noticed that neither of them wore combinations. My gratitude to the girl in the Co-op knew no bounds. I contemplated a lifetime of rheumatism with equanimity.

When both girls were decently covered in their flower-sprigged winceyette nightgowns I made a sort of tent with my dress and struggled to remove my underwear. When I found I was getting nowhere I quickly took off the dress and put the nightgown on over the rest of my clothes, then got into bed.

The red-headed girl was religious. Before she finally got into bed she knelt beside it and said her prayers. As she prayed she frequently kissed a small statue of a lady holding a little baby in her arms, and counted a string of beads between her fingers. Being brought up strictly Low Church I knew nothing about such visual aids to religion and could only assume she wore the beads as a keepsake from somebody, and kissed the lady to remind herself of her own dear mother probably dead. The pathos of the thought brought me round to the sadness of my own recent discoveries and I buried my head in the bedclothes and wept. I sniffled and choked for a long time before anybody took any notice of my sniffles. Then from one of the beds came a voice.

'You're new, aren't you? What's your name?' I took a deep breath, gave a last tremendous sniff and came up from the blankets. Then I spoke my real name aloud for the first time in my life. The moment I said it it sounded wrong and I waited for the girl to argue with me, but she didn't and I had crossed the first of many bridges my new identity was going to build for me.

Out of the darkness the other girl spoke. 'Did Mary tell you where the lavatory was? She nearly always forgets. One girl was here nearly a week before anybody told her, she almost burst.' Allowing for a margin of exaggeration I could imagine. Mary hadn't told me where the lavatory was either and it had been a long time since my mother warned me that the carrier's cart was just about due and I had better go round the back before he came.

I climbed out of bed and groped my way across the room. Neither of the girls spoke again and when I got back they were both asleep. Thankfully I took off the rest of my clothes, put my nightdress on again and went to bed. I tossed and turned for a full two minutes in the strange bed and woke to find someone shaking me violently and bawling something in my ear.

'Come on, wake up,' I heard them say. 'It's six o'clock and breakfast's at half-past. Sister will go mad if you're late. Then the cockerel in nurse's uniform rushed out of the room to do her crowing somewhere else.

The three of us dragged ourselves out of bed, took it in turns to have a quick rinse in a drop of cold water in a bowl in the corner and got into our uniforms. There was an urgency about it all that made me realize there was no time for niceties like turning my back to put my knickers on. The two girls fastened studs for me and fixed the cap on my head with Kirby grips they kindly lent me until I had some of my own. The list had said nothing about Kirby grips. When I was all dressed up I looked at myself in the dressing-table mirror and felt silly and self-conscious and wondered how long it would be before I could get a photograph taken to send to my mother.

Being now in full dress made me eligible for my share of the meal-time chores. I sat humbly at the foot of the table and got hot and flustered trying to obey every command that was directed at me. No allowance was made for my newness and I was soon in trouble for doing all the wrong things at all the wrong times. I fetched when I should have carried and brought when I should have taken. It was kippers for breakfast. My mother didn't believe in kippers any more than she believed in shrimps, so I had never come face to face with one in my life but the cries that rose from all around me left me in no doubt of their identity, however unfamiliar I was with their shape and smell.

'My God,' wailed every nurse with a single voice, 'not bloody kippers again, we had them yesterday.' Then they fell upon the kippers and ate them as if they had never eaten in their lives before. I was glad I was fully occupied tearing off slices of bread and chasing backwards and forwards to the hatch. One look at the kippers had been enough for me to realize that I would have needed more than the time allowed to cope with the bones. My mother's table etiquette hadn't taken care of things like kippers. It was a long time before I could eat one without instinctively dodging a clout.

When the last of the kipper plates with their interesting skeletons had reached my end of the table to be stacked in a pile ready to be taken to the hatch, a curious thing started happening. There was little more than five minutes left before we were due on the wards but suddenly every nurse grabbed her side plate and sat poised on the edge of her chair ready for flight. Then a maid appeared at the hatch door with a huge jar of marmalade. At once a surging mass of nurses – all thought of seniority forgotten – struggled and fought their way to the hatch to receive the tiny teaspoonful of marmalade the maid grudgingly apportioned out to them, then struggled and fought their way back to eat it.

There was no war on at the time, not in England anyway, nor any dearth of marmalade in the land, yet for as long as I was at the hospital the same ritual took place at the same time every morning. If the marmalade had been put on the table for us all to get at without a fight not nearly as much of it would have been eaten, but that would have been too easy and nothing was made easy for us, not even the dispensation of a teaspoonful of marmalade.

While the lucky ones who had reached the hatch before it was slammed shut in their face were enjoying the fruits of their chase there came a loud knocking from the sisters' table. They were given a whole jar of marmalade to themselves and had finished their breakfast with no unseemly haste. From the summit rose a sister as imposing as the home-sister was, with a bonnet just as lacy. She beat a tattoo on the table with a knife.

'Quiet please, Nurses,' she commanded in a ringing voice. Considering the instant hush that had fallen on the room from the moment she stood up, her command was unnecessary. All the senior sisters had to do to command hush was simply to be there, looking as if they wanted hush.

'Kindly listen carefully to what I am about to say.' We listened. You could have heard a pin drop. She waited until we were too intimidated even to cough, then she continued.

'As you all know, it is change day today.' She looked pointedly across at me. I was obviously the only one in the room unaware of the significance of change day. She gave me a second or two to recover from the news then she went on.

'All of you except the ones who are due for night duty will report to your new wards this morning. The change list on the notice board will tell you where you are to go. Those who are down for night duty will work on their previous wards until two o'clock, then move their things across to the night nurses' corridor and go to bed. They will be called for duty again this evening at eight o'clock. That will be all, Nurses. Kindly leave the mess-room quietly.' She sat down and bedlam broke out. Chairs fell, nurses pushed and maids swore. Everywhere was a confusion of feet and voices as each girl charged across the room to learn her fate. Wild shrieks and groans and mournful 'My Gods' filled the air. Nobody seemed happy at what they read. I stood alone, crushed and bewildered by it all. I had known nothing like it, not since wet days in the gymnasium at school, and even then the gym mistress was able to restore order before it got too out of hand. She had muscles like a prize fighter and a voice to match.

When the crowd had thinned out and there were only a few stragglers left behind I edged my way to the board and stretched and strained to find anything on it that might relate to me. There was no mention of the name that had been mine for the past eighteen years and so much had happened since the day before that I had already forgotten my new one. While I was still stretching and straining one of the stragglers noticed me and came across to me.

'Are you the new nurse?' she asked. I mulled over the question for a moment or two then realized that I must be. I nodded.

'Then for God's sake come on,' she screeched. 'We're

on Lavender's ward and we're late, she'll kill us.' She pushed me smartly in the middle of the back and we tore out of the mess-room. At last I was going to be a nurse.

Chapter Seven

WE BELTED DOWN corridors, across courtyards and along more corridors and slid to a standstill outside a ward door. We were late, as the nurse had predicted we would be, and the sister was standing at the door waiting to kill us. She was tall and slim and beautiful with a face that misled me into thinking she couldn't possibly be as awful as the nurse had warned me she was. I was soon to learn you can't always go by faces. When she saw us approaching she advanced towards us waving her arms in the air. She looked very menacing.

'And, just where do you two think you've been?' she stormed. Her voice hit the walls, ricocheted off them, echoed down the corridor and came back to us little the worse for its journey. There was a stridency about it that a regimental sergeant-major might have envied. I never heard it lowered by more than a decibel or two. Even when Lavender was being kind to a patient she screamed her compassion. She was never kind to us.

Lavender was not her real name. It had been bestowed upon her by a succession of nurses whose lives she had made miserable but who respected her even though they lived in terror of her. She was admired by everybody for her total dedication to her job, and feared by all for the way she did it. She was a born nurse, from her perfectly positioned cap to her mirror-bright shoes.

Still waving her arms about she went on raging. 'In future you will kindly remember to report on duty at the proper time, which is seven o'clock, not three minutes past. I will not have my nurses strolling on the ward just when it suits them.' Remembering our head-long chase down the corridors 'stroll' seemed hardly the right word to describe it. She looked furiously at the other nurse. 'You should know better than to be late on duty, get into the ward at once.' The nurse slunk off, glad to escape so lightly.

'And as for you,' said the sister, turning on me with renewed energy, 'I don't know where you were dragged up but you were obviously taught nothing at all about punctuality. Come into my office.' I followed her into her office, realizing that in one short sentence she had destroyed all the years of my mother's intensive training, yet I knew my mother would have thoroughly approved of her – they were quite definitely two of a kind.

For the next ten minutes I was treated to a harangue that covered a wide range of subjects: undeviating devotion to duty, strictest attention to detail, super-human physical endurance and absolute obedience to the wishes and commands of my seniors. At the end of it I was left in no doubt that the idea of me ever becoming a nurse was as ridiculous as my mother's dream of turning me into a lady. I was no more the right material for the one than I was for the other. The sister concluded with an ironic hope. 'If you have paid attention to what I've been telling you and work very hard we might be able to rub along together.'

'Yes, Miss – Sister,' I said, very much doubting it. She rang the bell for a nurse to come and remove me from her office. It was the same one who had conducted me there.

The ward we walked down looked cluttered and untidy to me but this was an optical illusion. Nothing was ever untidy on Lavender's ward, she never allowed it to be. The cluttered look was caused by there being several beds arranged down the middle of the ward as well as the twenty on either side. The nurse who was with me told me they were there because things were 'busy' at the moment. I never knew Lavender's ward when things were not 'busy'.

'It's a gynae ward,' went on the nurse. 'That means that all the women are in with something wrong with their wombs and things.' I blushed. It sounded rude to me. Where I came from wombs and things were not spoken of except in hushed voices.

At the far end of the ward there were a number of beds with rails round them. Most of the old women in them were stark naked. They were busily hanging their bedding and their nightdresses over the rails like washing hanging out to dry. They watched us suspiciously as we walked past them.

'I shouldn't take any notice of them if I were you,' said the nurse, seeing me staring at them. 'They are the poor old chronics. They've been in a long time and they're a bit barmy.' She spoke very kindly about them but I couldn't help thinking they were too old to expose themselves like that. I turned my head away.

When we reached the sluice which was to be my base for a long time, there was already a nurse working in there. I was surprised and delighted to see that it was one of the girls who slept in my room, the Welsh one, not the red-haired Irish girl. Her name was Davies and she came from Neath and had been to the same school as the film star Ray Milland which gave her the edge over me socially.

Despite the medical science she had tried to blind me with the night before while she was making her bed Davies had only been a nurse for three months and was still at the bedpan stage. She was as frightened about it all as she had been the day she started. Her mother was as strict as mine and used the same rule book to discipline her family by. Davies and I became firm friends and remained firm friends until we had both recovered enough from our uprootings to form other attachments, and even then we clung to each other in the face of the enemy. At Christmas and exam-results time, or whenever there were celebrations going on in the home that involved strong drink, we locked ourselves up in the bedroom and trembled. Neither of us was used to such celebrations and the thought of what might be going on right outside our door terrified us. She was perhaps more biased against the bottle than I was. My prejudices sprang from fear of the unknown; hers from deep religious principles – they are always hardest to combat. We were still as biased when we had finished our training.

The other girl in our room, being Irish, had no such inhibitions. She had been brought to screaming pitch at birth with a drop or two of whiskey and had never lost her taste for it. We were terrified of her as well, notwithstanding her beads and her statue. She told us that all her sisters were nuns and that she was going to be a nun after she had passed her finals, but we didn't believe her. Nuns were nuns, not flesh and blood girls like us. As it happened all her sisters *were* nuns, and her intention to be one was strictly honourable but she never became one. Instead she won a fantastic amount of money in a sweepstake and went off to America, but not, of course, until she had passed her finals.

When the nurse had gone and left us in the sluice Davies told me what I had to do. Having me there meant that I was the most junior nurse on the ward instead of her and she couldn't wait to use her new-found seniority. The promotion went to her head and made her very bossy with me.

'First you must hot the bedpans up under the tap ready for me to take them out. Sister doesn't allow us to give the patients cold bedpans. Then when I bring in the dirty ones you have to empty them and hot them up again.' I understood that the cycle would be repeated several times. She rushed off to gather in the first harvest.

As I took the bedpans from her and emptied the contents down the sink there went with them most of the romantic dreams of cool hands on fevered brows I had imagined nursing was all about. There had been no mention of bedpans in *Peg's Paper*. Only noble sacrifice and burning glances exchanged between doctors and nurses. I had to re-adjust my ideas quite a lot.

'You'd better do that one again,' said Davies throwing a reject back at me. 'The Matron looks down the handles when she does her round and she'll have you in the office if she finds a dirty one.'

While I was poking down the handles to make them fit for the Matron to look through I had a sudden vision of her view being obstructed by a wad of some indescribable filth and I bent down to have a good giggle. Unfortunately in doing so I knocked against a lever which released a jet of water that shot to the ceiling and fell at my feet in a Niagara-like deluge. I stood rooted to the spot getting wetter all the time. Luckily Davies came in with a pile of bedpans which she promptly dropped. Then she fell upon the lever and turned it off. We stood dripping and giggling in the puddles and it began to seem as if nursing was going to have its lighter side after all. Our hilarity did not last long. Attracted by the clatter of falling bedpans a ward maid rushed in to find out what had happened. She took one look at us and at the mess on the floor said, 'Oh my God,' and rushed off to fetch the sister. The sister was busy with something else so the staff-nurse came and dealt with us. She made an excellent job of it and by the time she had finished with us neither Davies nor I was giggling. We cleared up the mess in silence, each of us pondering over the unkind things the staff-nurse had said about us. I had the added burden of feeling responsible for Davies's downfall.

If scraping out the bedpans had done nothing to foster the romance of nursing the next two hours we spent in the ward were just as uninspiring. While our seniors rushed about giving medicines and injections, arranging fallen pillows and doing unimaginable things behind screens, Davies and I sweated and slaved pulling beds out into the centre of the ward and sweeping, buffing and polishing every inch of floor space. When it was all gleaming we started on the beds. 'We have to polish the springs,' said Davies. 'When the Matron does her round, she brings a walking stick with her and picks up the sides of the mattresses. If she finds any dust on the springs we'll both be in her office tomorrow morning.' We polished the springs until they shone, pushing the patients this way and that regardless of their post-operative groans.

While we worked the staff-nurse kept us under constant surveillance, carping and criticizing and spurring us on to ever greater breathless endeavour. It was as much in Lavender's interest as it was in ours to see that the Matron's fingers were as lily white when she finished the round as they were when she started. Unless they were we got a black mark in our ward report and some doubt was expressed about Lavender's ability to train us properly. Hence the staff-nurse's unflagging interest in our activities.

When the dirtiest of the ward work had been done and the spurring and goading failed to produce any better results we were allowed to go across to the home to have our lunch and change our aprons. 'Lunch' was a meal like my father's snap but less plentiful. Slabs of bread and dripping or cheese, and cups of nasty cocoa were laid out for us in the mess-room and we got through as much of it as we could in the shortest possible time then rushed up to our rooms to change our aprons and make our beds ready for Mary to come and strip them again. When it was all done Davies looked at her watch.

'If we hurry, we'll just have time to go to the library for a cigarette.' I stared at her. With her strict upbringing coupled with religion I had certainly not expected her to have vices like smoking.

'I don't smoke,' I told her a little smugly.

'You will,' she said. 'I didn't when I first came here. My mam would have a fit if she knew.' And so would mine I thought as we slammed the door behind us.

The library was a box-like room without a book in sight. Neither was there a carpet on the floor, any chairs to sit on or curtains at the window. This marked lack of hospitality was the Matron's way of telling her nurses that though she had moved with the times enough to allow them to smoke, they were not to run away with the idea that she approved of the habit. Her implied disapproval did nothing to stop her nurses standing about in cliquey groups drawing frantically at their cigarettes in a desperate attempt to get through as many as possible before it was time to go back on duty.

I stood with Davies inside the smoky circle until she almost burnt her fingers on the stub then we went back to the ward. In less than thirty minutes we had eaten a substantial meal, made our beds after a fashion, changed our aprons and stuffed everything out of sight in the bedroom, and stood about in the library long enough for Davies to calm her jangled nerves with a cigarette.

We crept silently past Lavender's office and had just broken into a run at the last lap when she came out onto the corridor.

'Nurses,' she shouted. We stopped in our tracks. 'Come back at once.' We went back. 'Did I hear you running?' Davies and I looked at each other. With the office door tightly shut it was unlikely that she would have heard us running.

'No, Sister,' we said hopefully. She couldn't have heard us running. She looked from one to the other of us and finally decided to believe us.

'Don't ever let me find you running,' she said severely. 'This is a hospital not a sports stadium. The only time a nurse is allowed to run is in cases of fire or haemorrhage and even then a good nurse will proceed in an orderly fashion without showing signs of panic.' She glared at us.

'Yes, Sister,' we said and were just starting back on our journey into the ward when she called me. 'I'll see you in my office,' she said. I cringed. I was still smarting from the morning interview with her in her office.

She ran her eyes over my cap, my apron, my shoes and stockings, took in the faults, registered them for future reference then sat back in her chair and began her second lecture of the day.

'I suppose you want to know about your off-duty,' she began. 'It's all you nurses ever seem to think about, though in my opinion probationers are pampered enough already without getting off-duty as well. You'll get two hours off a day when I can spare you, a half-day a week and a day off a month, but don't start thinking you've got a right to it. If we're busy you won't get any. I can't run a ward without nurses and when I did my training nurses were glad enough to stay on duty for ever if the need arose.' She gave me another furious look and I stumbled out of the office. Everything she had said was true. She was a dedicated nurse and would certainly have stayed on duty for ever if the need arose, and expected the same dedication from her staff. She was often disappointed.

Every Monday morning a list had to be sent to the Matron's office giving precise details of all the off-duty for the week. Lavender dutifully sent in her list then forgot about it. Nobody but herself was allowed to see the duplicate list she kept locked up in a drawer in her office. Two minutes before she decided we were to go off she would send for us. With a look of one making the supreme sacrifice, and as if she were bestowing a tremendous favour on us, she would admit us into the office where we stood nervously wondering what was in store for us. 'You can go off duty, Nurse, but see that you're back in time. It's bad enough having to be without staff without them taking advantage and being late back.' And we would leave the ward with a tremendous feeling of guilt that we were failing in our duty by going at all.

This total lack of foreknowledge made any planning of a social life impossible and lost us many a boyfriend. However besotted they may have been before, they soon lost interest when we went on Gynae and could no longer tell them with any certainty when we were likely to be available.

As well as grudging us our off-duty, Lavender grudged us our meal-times. She often forgot to send us to the mess-room until it was too late to get anything to eat, and then blamed us for not getting there sooner.

'You'd better get across for your dinner,' she would scream from one end of the ward to the other. 'And don't spend all day eating it.'

'Please, Sister, it's too late.'

'You've got a tongue in your head, haven't you? Why couldn't you have asked to go at the proper time?' It would have been more than our lives were worth.

Davies and I missed more meals than the other nurses on the ward through these lapses of memory. Closeted as we were in the sluice we were easily forgotten. Luckily Davies had learned a trick or two during her short spell at the hospital. She passed on her tips to me.

'All you have to do is wait until Lavender and the staff-nurse go into the office for their after-dinner cup of tea then we can take it in turns to stand behind the kitchen door and eat what's left of the patients' dinners.' What was left of the patients' dinners was usually cold boiled cod and spotted dick, none of which went down very well with the patients, but they went down very well with us when we were hungry, and we were always hungry. The other nurses turned a blind eye, but we had to watch out for the ward maids during these alfresco meals. If one of them caught us stuffing the cod in our mouths and was in a bad temper, she would rush at once to the office and report us to Lavender who was duty bound to send us to the Matron in the morning. There were no laws against us missing our meals but there were plenty against us eating on the ward. It would have been useless for us to defend ourselves by pleading hunger.

The ward maids were monsters to be feared. Most of them had been at the hospital a long time and had established their position. They were the sisters' confidantes and kept them informed of anything that might have escaped them, and were rewarded for their spying with small privileges which put them above the nurses. If it had come to the point where either a nurse or a ward maid had to be boiled in oil it would have been the nurse who got popped in the pot. We all knew this and went out of our way to keep the ward maids happy.

Missing tea was never as dangerous as missing our dinner. If we were on duty in the afternoon we spent most of it cutting innumerable slices of bread for the patients' tea and pouring on them the liquid margarine we had forgotten to rescue from the hot-plate where it had been put to soften. While we were stacking up the bread it was a simple matter to dodge the maids and stuff ourselves with slices on the side. Doing it this way we managed to get cake once or twice a week. We hardly ever got cake in the mess-room, and when we did there was never enough to go round, or, like the marmalade, it only made its appearance when it was too late to get any pleasure from it.

When the hospital became a training school for male nurses, an extra table was put up for them next to the sisters and they got buns every day. We never got buns. It was long before our time that a Mrs Pankhurst chained herself to the railings to win for women a fair share of what the men had. As far as we were concerned she might as well have stayed safely at home in her drawing-room. We never got a fair share of what the men had. It was for this reason and this reason alone that we regarded the first lot of male nurses with deep suspicion. It took us a long time to get used to them. Some of us never did get used to them.

When Lavender had finished explaining her off-duty system to me I went up to the sluice for Davies to tell me what I had to do next. She was standing knee-deep in dirty washing. She gave me a warning frown and went on counting.

'Forty draw sheets, thirty top sheets, sixty pillow slips, what do you want?'

'What do I do next?' I asked her, trying to sound as if I wasn't there at all. She raised her eyes to heaven in an exasperated way and went on with the washing. When she had come to the last towel she looked at me and thought deeply. Suddenly her eyes lit up.

'You can clean the lavatories,' she said, sounding very pleased about it. Until that day it had been her job to clean the lavatories but now that she was second probationer she could move up to doing the bathroom taps instead, which was a distinct improvement. Anything was an improvement on cleaning the lavatories.

It was while I was half in and half out of a lavatory pan trying to get at the U-bend that the Matron arrived on her tour of Inspection. She pushed open the door. I stood smartly to attention, banged my head on the window ledge and fell back in a sitting position on the lavatory seat. She looked at me in mild surprise. I stared back at her from my lowly position.

'What on earth are you sitting there for, Nurse?' she asked. Lavender craned her neck to see what was going on and after a muttered explanation about me being new that day they passed on. I sat for a moment on the seat to get my breath back before attacking the U-bend again.

When the sluices, lavatories and bathrooms were as clean as Davies and I could make them we went into the ward to help the seniors get everything ready for visiting day. Sunday was visiting day and a lot of preparation had to be made for it. Clean nightdresses were put on, hair brushed, sheets smoothed, lockers tidied, stools put out for the visitors to sit on, chronics bawled out and warned to keep their clothes on while the visitors were there, and every patient was threatened what Sister would say if they didn't keep themselves and their beds tidy until two o'clock when visiting day officially started. Officially, because Lavender had her own way of organizing visiting days.

The time allowed was two hours but this was cut considerably by Lavender standing on guard outside the ward door keeping everybody waiting while she vetted each visitor for their right to enter. However near and dear they were to the patient they had to stand while she made a quick appraisal of their age (nobody was admitted under the age of sixteen), their relationship to the patient (two husbands arriving simultaneously to visit one wife could cause a lot of embarrassment), but above all the physical condition they were in. This was checked assiduously. A drunk had got into the ward once without anybody spotting him. The results were apparently riveting. He had been deprived of his home comforts for a long time and was set on finding out what, if any, improvements the surgeon had made on his future conjugal rights. Lavender was determined that nothing like this should happen again. And it never did.

As well as keeping constant vigil herself outside the ward door Lavender kept every nurse who was on duty busily employed at vantage points inside the ward. To the casual observer they were innocently turning out medicine cupboards, doing something to one of the grannies behind a screen, or stripping and re-stripping the cot-beds at the end of the ward. The poor old chronics seldom got any visitors so were an ideal cover for the secret-agent work which went on to keep the visiting side in order. Should one of them be wicked enough to rest his backside for a moment on the clean white counterpane put on specially for the day, or be undisciplined enough to smuggle in a portion of forbidden food, the spies fell over themselves to report the culprit to the sister, who, after laying the law down and threatening the offender with expulsion if he ever sinned again, complimented the 'grass' on her powers of observation and promised to mention her in the ward report at the end of the month.

Powers of observation were highly esteemed in the profession. Without them, we were told, we could never hope to reach the heights. With them we could get almost anywhere. A word in the right ear about something we had observed being done in the wrong way at the wrong time was enough to earn us the approval of many of our seniors, but not with Lavender, except where the visitors were concerned and they didn't really matter; they were on the other side of the counter. Lavender was loyal to her staff and only listened to the tales that the ward maids carried, and even then she had to see for herself before she took any action, but like the home-sister she seldom missed anything.

After all the hard work I had done to get ready for it I was robbed of the thrills of that first visiting day. A few minutes before second dinner was over the staff-nurse came down to the sluice where I was getting the bedpans ready for the after-dinner round. She took the one I was currently running under the hot tap, glued the handle to her eye and looked down it. Much to her disappointment it was clean. She flung it back at me and spoke angrily.

'Sister says you can go off for the afternoon. You'd better go to dinner and come back again after first tea. And see you're back prompt, we don't want any repeats of this morning.' She flounced off. Within seconds she was back. 'Well, what are you standing there for, you'll be late for dinner, then blame Sister. Roll your sleeves down, put your cuffs on and go and ask her if you can go to dinner.' I did as I was told and knocked at the office door.

'Please may I go to dinner?' I asked timidly.

'I suppose so,' said Lavender ungraciously. I got to the mess- room just as the first course dishes were being collected and scraped. The maids looked daggers at me as I slunk to my seat.

'I suppose you're from Gynae,' said one of them sulkily. 'Why that Lavender can't send you for your dinners at the proper time I'll never know.' She opened the hatch and stuck her head inside. I could hear her yelling to somebody in the distance and after a long time she came back and thrust a plate in front of me. On it was the first Sunday dinner I had ever eaten that my mother hadn't had a hand in cooking.

Chapter Eight

THE SUNDAY DINNERS we ate in our house had been the combined efforts of my father and my mother. On Saturday afternoon my mother roasted the joint, de-caterpillared the greens, peeled the potatoes and beat the batter for the Yorkshire pudding until it sounded like a cavalry of horses galloping up the cart-track. None of this was done in obedience to the fourth commandment but in order that we should be sitting safely in our pews at church when the last bell rang out on Sunday morning.

Before we went off to church, and after my father had put a bit of air in our bicycle tyres, my mother led him on a conducted tour of the larder. She took the lids off the saucepans and showed him their contents, telling him the exact moment when they should be put on the hob to start simmering. She introduced him to the Yorkshire pudding, already in a dripping tin with a rim of congealed fat round the edge, and reminded him to put it in a brisk oven no later than twelve and keep the fire well stoked up so that the pudding would be risen to a mountainous perfection by the time we got home, ready to be eaten soaked in gravy before our main course.

My father was proud of his Yorkshire puddings and took all the credit for their lightness and crispness. He never would admit that my mother's beating and the length of the vicar's sermon had anything to do with their perfection. Neither would he have recognized the flat square of soggy dough that lay on my plate flanked by a slice of stringy meat, two spoonfuls of wet cabbage and some black shells of over-roast potatoes. The piece of pie I was given afterwards bore even less resemblance to my mother's cooking. It floated in a liquid that I realized was custard-powder custard. I thought it tasted far inferior to ours but that could have been because of the way the hospital cooks had put the ingredients together. It is an indisputable fact that, given exactly the same set of ingredients, the same working conditions and the same recipe, hospital cooks invariably produce something that tastes entirely different from everybody else's product. I ate the dinner to the last drop, then flagrantly disobeying the home-sister's warnings, I went across to my room. The three beds were stripped but not to the springs. It was Sunday and even Mary drew the line at removing mattresses on Sundays. I left the bedding on the floor, drew my long black cape around me and threw myself on the bed. Within seconds I was asleep and within seconds I was awake again. Mary had observed my entry into the room, waited for my exit and not seeing one had come to investigate. Her voice cut through the weight of weariness that was pinning down my eyelids.

'Really, Nurse, this is disgraceful. I thought I told you yesterday that I didn't allow any sitting about in your rooms. And here you are actually lying asleep on your bed. Get up at once, make your bed and go down to the sitting-room. You know where the sitting-room is, don't you?'

I prised my eyes open and threw my aching feet over the edge of the bed. 'Yes, Sister,' I said.

'Only here a day and already breaking the rules,' she grumbled, and went.

The sitting-room was a long narrow room with a lot of uncomfortable-looking leather chairs and sofas lining the walls. The springs sprang out of them everywhere. Like the nettles round our back they would need to be carefully arranged before comfort could be assured.

At each end of the room there was a mock-Adam fireplace. Only rarely did a fire burn in either of them. The weather had to reach Arctic conditions before Mary would give her consent to such wild extravagance. When the temperature was at normal freezing point we kept ourselves warm by drawing our feet up under our capes and keeping our ears buried under the hood.

As well as the chairs, sofas and fireplaces there was a wireless set and a pianola that had been donated to us by a friendly Friendly Society. None of us ever saw the pianola in action. It turned out later there should have been some sort of rolls with holes in – we never saw them either.

If the chairs and sofas in the sitting-room offered little comfort for our tortured bodies, other blessings could often be found concealed within their chilly depths. By plunging our hands deep down in their sagging sides we could sometimes come up with enough small change to buy a packet of Woodbines or Park Drives. Though not the ultimate in cigarette luxury – at twopence for five we were only too glad of them when funds were low at the end of the month. The brand we favoured most not only gave us a nasty hacking cough but had an extra 'four for your friends' stuck down the outside of the packet at no added cost. The bonus came in very handy for bribing the lodge-men with.

I spent my afternoon off dozing fitfully in one of the chairs and woke up in a panic too late to go to tea. I bundled my hair back in the cap, clamped it securely with grips and hurried back to the ward. The staff-nurse was waiting for me. She was in charge and looked as hot and bothered as I was.

'You're late,' she said untruthfully. I apologized.

'You can thank your lucky stars Sister's not on. She's had just about enough of you today, what with coming on duty late this morning, dropping bedpans all over the place and sitting on the lavatory while the Matron was talking to you. Which reminds me, the Matron wants to see you in her office tomorrow morning.'

I wilted. 'Was it something I did?' I asked cravenly. She let me sweat for a few minutes before she answered. She was notorious for her sadism.

'No, though considering the things you did it could just have been. As it happens she sees all new nurses on Monday morning. So mind you put a clean cap on and scrape your hair back a bit. She doesn't like seeing hair all over the place.' With this in mind I struggled through the rest of the day.

The evening was worse than the morning had been. Davies had been given a much coveted evening off which meant that I was not only the most junior nurse on duty but the second most junior as well. As well as emptying the bedpans, scouring them and hotting them up, I had to rush in and out of the ward with them while the third-year nurse who was putting the patients on them told me off for idling my time away in the sluice. Third-year nurses were always irritable when they were called upon to do anything with bedpans. Bedpans were beneath their dignity, but with Davies off and me too inexperienced to place a patient on a bedpan there was nothing the third-year nurse could do about it except vent her anger on me, which she did without cease.

'Don't you know how to clean a bedpan properly?' she fumed.

'Yes, Nurse,' I said.

'Then for God's sake why don't you clean them properly?' I cleaned the next one properly, only to find her standing behind me in the sluice.

'For God's sake what are you messing about at? It doesn't take all night to clean a bedpan does it?'

'No, Nurse,' I admitted, leaving the handle clogged up with tow.

When the bedpan round was over we started something that was called 'doing the backs'. Again because of Davies being off I was called in to assist.

'Bring the screens,' ordered the third-year nurse. I dragged two heavy iron screens the full length of the ward and arranged them round the bed she indicated. Then I stood and waited. The third-year nurse stood and waited as well.

'Well, where's the trolley and the dirty linen bin?' she asked. I didn't know but I was too frightened to say so.

'How am I expected to do the backs with no trolley and no dirty linen bin?' she inquired reasonably. She still stood and waited while I went back to the sluice and located both the required pieces of equipment.

'Now get to the other side of the bed,' she demanded. I looked at her with my mouth open. What I was expected to do when I got to the other side of the bed was something I couldn't even guess at.

'Don't stand there gaping like an idiot,' she said. 'Help me to turn the patient over and hold her while I do her back.' I did as I was told. I clutched the patient to my bosom and held her while the nurse on the other side of the bed scoured the portion of anatomy that was offered to her with a mixture of soap and water, methylated spirits and a generous helping of elbow grease. I kept expecting the patient to protest at the invasion of her modesty but she didn't. Instead, when we had finished she gave a blissful sigh.

'Eeh, that was fair grand, duck, its luvly to get your back done.' She looked up at me gratefully.

'It's your first day isn't it, duck?' I nodded. 'Never mind, you'll get used to it after a bit, won't she, Nurse?' The nurse smiled and patted her hand. We straightened the bed, shook the pillows and sat the patient comfortably amongst them and I got the first germ of an idea that some day it might be quite satisfying to be a nurse. The day wasn't too long dawning.

When the last back had been 'done', the last screen returned to base and the bins and trolleys cleared up I went into the sluice and got on with the laundry. Getting on with the laundry was a very unpleasant business. It was not simply a matter of counting pillow cases. Some of the ladies in the cot beds were not too particular about their personal habits and it was my duty to see that the sheets off their beds were without stain when the porters came to collect them. The porters were fussy about what they would handle and if there was something they didn't like the look of they either dragged it up the ward and waved it under the nose of whoever was in charge or left it behind and sent the head porter to the Matron to do their complaining for them. I was still doing my best to ensure that the sheets were pure enough to suit the most fastidious porter when the staff-nurse came storming in like a whirlwind.

'For goodness' sake, Nurse, stop wasting your time in here and get to the kitchen and wash the supper things up.' Washing up the supper things was the ward maid's work, but if the ward maid was off or didn't feel like doing the washing up it fell to the junior nurse to do it. I dragged myself up the ward.

When I got to the kitchen and saw the mountain of washing up my heart sank. I scraped the plates and filled the sink. Just as I was about to plunge my arms into the greasy water two women came to the door. They were both in their nightdresses. They looked at me and at the stack of dishes, then at each other. They were both fat and jolly looking. They rolled up the sleeves of their nightdresses and pushed me out of the way.

'Don't you worry about this lot, duck. We'll soon get rid of it for you won't we, Doll?'

'That we will, Lizzy,' said Doll. 'It's not fair expecting her to do it all and on her first day at that.' I looked at them gratefully then an awful thought struck me.

'But what will she say if she comes in?' I asked.

'What will who say?' asked Doll.

'The staff-nurse,' I said, looking fearfully at the door.

'Oh never you mind about her,' said Lizzy. 'She'll not be back this side of seven. She's buggered off next door for a cup of tea. It's a case of when the cat's away the mice will play. It's more than she dare do if the sister was on duty, isn't it, Doll?'

'That's right, Lizzy,' said Doll. 'If she comes back and starts giving us any of her lip we'll soon tell her to go to hell.' Lizzy washed while Doll dried. I put the things away without the least idea of where they should go.

'Me and Doll's going to the theatre tomorrow,' said Lizzy. 'We're going to have our insides took out.' I looked at her in amazement. How would they live with their insides out and how could they look so happy about it? Doll must have read my thoughts. She put a broken cup with all the other breakages and went on.

'It's about time they took my lot out,' she said cheerfully. 'The doctor told me after me last miss that if I fell again it would be the end of me. But it's not a bit of good talking to my George, he doesn't take no notice. He's always the same when he's had a drop too much.' I was mystified by the talk. What had Doll missed, and where was she expecting to fall from? And what was her George the same about when he'd had a drop too much? The questions screamed to be asked but I was too polite to ask them. All I could do was listen.

'I know what you mean,' sympathized Lizzy. 'We could have done wi'out our Sally but nowt shifted her. The woman next door offered to do it for me but the last one she did for me went septic so my Jack wouldn't let her touch me this time.' She threw a few more pots into the sink. 'I went to that herbalist down Mansfield Road once but he's as mucky as her next door to me. He never washes his hands and his place is filthy. He's in prison now and serve him right an' all.'

The women finished the washing up and I thanked them for doing it for me. I could just as easily have thanked them for giving me something to think about for the rest of that weary evening. But however much I puzzled over what I had heard I could make neither head nor tail of it, though it wouldn't be long before I did.

When I got back to the ward after I had been for my own supper, everywhere was a buzz of activity. The nurses were flying about as if they were expecting royalty. 'We're getting ready for the night nurses coming on,' called out third-year, charging past me with a sweeping brush in her hand. Fourth-year was rushing about whisking flowers away while the staff-nurse stood at the door issuing orders. 'Hurry up and get ready for the night nurses,' she screamed when she saw me.

Getting ready for the night nurses meant doing again most of the things that had been done twice already that evening. Floors were swept, lockers dusted, beds straightened and the furbished re-furbished. Everywhere was restored from perfect order to even more perfect order. The patients were lifted up, laid down, turned over and turned back again, until they were exactly where they were before but a lot less comfortable. The chronics were put into their nightdresses for the dozenth time. The night nurses came on at nine and unless everything was in faultless condition when they arrived, they complained to the night sister who complained to the day sister who defended her honour by taking the complaint to the Matron. A permanent battle raged between the two shifts with the probationers the casualties on both sides. It was of vital importance to them to make sure the war never got as far as the Matron's office. It was to that end that the final hour of the outgoing staff was spent in feverish activity getting ready for the incoming staff.

A few minutes before nine o'clock the staff-nurse sent for us.

'Is everything ready for the night staff?' she asked anxiously. We assured her it was. Not satisfied she went over everything herself. She rubbed her fingers over the lockers, sniffed the water in the jugs to make sure it had been renewed, stripped a sheet back at random to see that the bottom one was unruffled, inspected the sluices, bathrooms, lavatories, rubbish bins, linen bins and pig bins and finally admitted that everything was indeed ready for the night staff. We breathed again. She looked at me.

'All right you can go now, and don't forget what I told you about putting a clean cap on and scraping your hair back for the Matron in the morning.'

'No, Nurse. Thank you, Nurse,' I said gratefully and went off duty.

Davies was already in bed and asleep when the Irish girl and I went into the room. We crept about so as not to waken her. We knew only too well how valuable sleep had become. The Irish girl did her thing with her beads and then turned out the light. As I stretched my throbbing feet to the bottom of the bed I remembered with surprise that it was still only Sunday, and little more than a day had passed since I was a girl at home

with only my mother to scream at my wrongdoings. I
fell asleep thinking of the visit to the Matron that the
staff-nurse had promised me.

Chapter Nine

GOING TO THE Matron was something we did often, especially in the first year or two of our training. The visits were never social calls, neither did they leave behind many happy memories. All it took to send us shivering with apprehension to the office at ten o'clock in the morning was a shattered thermometer, dropped carelessly and with intent to rob the hospital of a valuable piece of equipment, a less than gleaming bath tap, a complaint from Mary that our bed hadn't been made properly for yet a second time that week or a report from a gate-porter – who had refused to perjure his soul for a packet of Park Drives – that we had booked in a split second after ten instead of on the dot on our evening off. All were heinous crimes and punishable by the disgrace and terror of being sent to the Matron.

Despite the warnings I got from Davies and the Irish girl while they were making up a clean cap for me and shoving each whisker of hair inside it so that none should escape to offend the Matron's eye my first visit was worse than anything I could have anticipated.

On Monday morning I stood outside the office door with all the other suspects and known criminals. Some shook visibly, others more experienced in sin and its consequences tried to look nonchalant, but all around us there was a smell of sweat oozing from nervous pores that made the corridor a nasty place to be in at ten o'clock in the morning. We all shuffled guiltily from one foot to the other. Nurses without a stain on their characters passed by with a sanctimonious sneer; less saintly ones looked the other way knowing that, but for the grace of God and a little extra cunning, they could have been standing there themselves.

When it came to my turn and the sharp command to enter rang out in answer to my timid knock, I flung open the door in nervous reflex, missed the step that both Davies and the Irish girl had warned me about and fell headlong into the room. The fat Scottie dog they had also mentioned in passing came panting across the room and threw himself upon my recumbent body. Playfully he tore off my cap and was already gnawing at my shoes before I managed to push him away. The Matron sat at her desk and watched with a look of weary resignation on her face. She had obviously seen it all before.

Mercifully the dog was old and wheezy and soon lost interest in me. He waddled across the room with my cap in his mouth and I struggled to a vertical position. Getting the cap out of the dog's mouth took several minutes but at last it was back on my head and I stood smartly to attention at the Matron's desk waiting for her to open the conversation. She took her time. She looked me up and down for a long while before she said anything. When she spoke her voice was very unfriendly.

'And how, may I ask, do you expect to deal with the lives of your patients if you are unable to come into a room without making a fool of yourself?' How indeed? She went on looking at me and I squirmed beneath her look. She was a stout lady, firmly corseted and with a bust-line that clearly indicated she was wearing the pink brioche bodices the village shop had specialized in. She had tremendous presence and an air of calm that never deserted her. The nurse who went into her office many years later and found her sitting at her desk quite dead was rumoured to have said she looked no different then than she had any other morning. We believed the rumour. It would have taken more than death to ruffle the Matron's calm. She stirred no emotions in us other than fear. Nobody ever said, 'Isn't the Matron nice?' or, 'Isn't the Matron nasty?' She was the Matron and above such earthly judgement. There was a sister who was heard referring to her as 'The Old Cream Bun'. Her nurses shrank from her for weeks, certain that the hand of God would strike her down for such blasphemy. It never did. The hand of God never seems as ready to strike down as the hot gospellers would have us believe. My mother was a case in point. She didn't believe in sewing on Sunday. If a button came off, or a vital piece of elastic snapped anywhere between Saturday night and Monday morning my mother took a needle and thread and concealed herself behind the living-room door to do the running repairs, presumably so that the Almighty wouldn't catch her at it. If he did he must have turned a blind eye or was in a good mood at the time. She was never struck down, and in fact she lived to a ripe old age.

The conversation I had with the Matron was as one-sided as the conversation with Lavender had been the morning before and ran on much the same lines though in even greater depth. When I emerged from the office I was discouraged and defeated, and wondered, as I was to wonder many times during the next three years, how my mother could have deluded herself into thinking I would ever find fame as a Nightingale. The Matron had clearly wondered the same thing.

I returned to the ward with my stomach rumbling with emptiness. Going to the Matron had left no time for going to the mess-room and I missed my bread and dripping and cocoa. Contrary to the bitter memory of the day before, Sunday had been a day of rest after all. On Monday life began in earnest and the spurring and goading were doubly intensified. When I went to tell Lavender I was back she turned on me savagely. 'And about time too,' she screamed. 'Idling your time away in the Matron's office while all the work is being done. Go to the staff-nurse and find out what your special duties are for the day, and be quick about it, you've wasted enough valuable time already.'

'Yes, Sister,' I said, conscious of the disruption my absence must have created on the ward. I wandered about looking for the staff-nurse.

As well as the scouring of floors, furniture, bedpans and the patients' bottoms that had sent me limping to my bed the night before, on all other days except Sundays we were allotted special duties. These included washing down walls wherever there was a wall to be washed, scrubbing out lockers and cupboards already snowy white from their previous scrubbing, and scraping the fluff and other adhesions from the wheels and castors of all movable apparatus in order to make them more easily moved. The beds were included in this category. If the nurse who had done them before had been less than conscientious there was often only one wheel that went round properly, which made sweeping beneath the beds harder work than it was already. Davies had been advised by those who had moved on to higher things to use a cloth soaked in ether meth for removing the more stubborn clingings. The practice was both dangerous and illegal but every junior did it. We did anything that looked like making things a bit easier for us however illegal or dangerous it may have been. One day, when we had searched everywhere for Davies to tell her that Lavender was looking for her, we found her snoring gently behind a screen, anaesthetized with the fumes from the ether meth. She looked so peaceful lying there it seemed a pity to waken her.

I found the staff-nurse and she stood weighing me up for a while before she made up her mind about my capabilities.

'You'd better do the bathroom walls first, and mind you do them properly. Then if there's any time left before we start the dinners you can help nurse Davies with the knitting.' Banished to the bathroom I was filled with envy at the thought of Davies being assigned to the knitting. I was wrong. Monday was nit day. On Monday mornings every junior nurse on every female ward longed to be given the job of nitting. There was an importance about getting a tray ready and going through the patients' heads with a small-toothed comb and swabs of sassafras oil that surpassed anything we did in the way of nursing for our first six months at least. The result of the hunt was carefully recorded in the head book and sent to the Matron each week with the back book, the bath book and all the other books tracking our attention to detail and powers of observation. If there was a head on one of the women that refused to come clean the Matron came herself or sent one of her deputies to check and re-check until all life was extinct. No patient was allowed to go out with the same nits she came in with.

We did the job thoroughly, cracking each nit noisily and triumphantly. If we were lucky enough to find a real live louse scurrying about among the Marcel waves we held it up between our thumb and finger and showed it round. The patients were never as happy at the find as we were.

One of the daily special duties was doing the teeth. This was a much less sought-after occupation. Removing and scrubbing the dentures belonging to anybody unable to remove and scrub their own was a job that had to be foisted on someone else wherever it was possible. Being last in line for the foisting I was usually left doing the teeth. The first time it happened and the staff-nurse told me to do the teeth and be quick about it I misinterpreted her instructions. I collected all the dentures from the chronics at the end of the ward, threw them into a bowl and cleaned them as they had never been cleaned before. The poor old grannies were to suffer many an attack of acute gastric disturbance before all the mistakes could be rectified. Sorting out one set of false teeth from another isn't easy – they have too many things in common.

I was in the bathroom, balancing on a pair of step ladders with a bucket, a scrubbing brush and a bar of Monkey Brand soap when Davies rushed in the door. She knocked against the ladder, dislodging the bucket and sending its scummy contents pouring down the half of the wall I had already cleaned.

'You'd better get down off there,' she said, picking her way through the scum and not bothering to apologize. 'It's nearly time for the doctor's round and we all have to be in the ward when he gets here.' I followed the bucket down the steps. Davies shrieked with alarm when I was on terra firma.

'My God,' she said. 'You'd better not let Lavender see you looking like that, she'll go mad. You've got water running down your arms and your cap's nearly off. It's Mr John's day and we have to be spotless when he comes, he's very particular.' We did a quick clean-up job on me and then went into the ward and stood in line for Lavender to find our faults before Mr John noticed them. There only had to be a button undone for him to jump on the offending nurse. He wasn't the only one who was particular. All the eminences that visited the ward were particular. The pomp and circumstance that surrounded their visit rose and fell according to their importance in the medical world. They were usually men. Lady doctors still hadn't caught on much and even if one did pay us a visit, she was never given the worshipping welcome we showered on her male colleagues and they accepted as their right. Female doctors, like male nurses, were something we had to get used to. It took a long time.

The arrival of the Illustrious One was heralded by a drum-roll of warning telephone calls from the places he had just left, and by the time he appeared at the door with his following of acolytes, satellites and right-hand men every nurse had abandoned whatever she was doing, except the most urgent, and was standing to attention with her sleeves rolled down, her cuffs on, her hair scraped back and her apron smoothed, ready to walk in solemn procession and in the strictest order of seniority behind the august personage. While the round was in progress all normal living came to a standstill. No books were read lest the rustle of leaves should disturb the hallowed hush, no drinks were drunk, no water passed and no bowels opened, except down among the chronics where things went on as if nothing was happening. They wouldn't have stopped taking their nightdresses off for Angel Gabriel himself.

As the tour progressed from bed to bed we listened in rapt awe to the jargon that fell from the sacred lips. Only the sister was fully aware of what he was talking about. She was so well up in it all that as soon as the round was over the lesser of the right-hand men went into her office to have their mistakes put right over coffee and biscuits before they did irreparable damage to someone with their misunderstandings, or went about ordering opening medicines instead of closing ones and vice versa.

If the round took longer than usual the trolley with the ward dinners in it was left standing where the porters had left it, the food getting colder every minute. Luckily for us, most of the patients were too stunned by what the surgeon had told them to notice what they were eating, so we were able to dish out the cold food without too many complaints. The surgeon's round on the Gynae ward was never without drama. The Gynae ward was never without drama either.

We were no more than eighteen when we started our training but from the moment we got into uniform we became ageless and sexless. The women on Lavender's ward regarded us all as their contemporaries. They told us dirty stories and let us into fascinating secrets of their married life which they would have hesitated to tell their sisters or their own mothers, let alone their eighteen-year-old daughters. At first we listened and blushed though not understanding half they were telling us, but soon we were throwing in comments of our own, only slightly less crude and as little informed as theirs were. We learned to laugh at things that had been veiled in delicacy and mystery before and it began to dawn on me that Brian's disclosures in the choir stalls might be nearer to the truth than *Peg's Paper*'s romantic version. With their light-hearted treatment of sex the women made it sound almost believable. Except for my parents and the vicar of course.

But if the quality of the wit was low there was no shortage of high tragedy on the Gynae ward. Twice a week a procession of trolleys wound its way to the main theatre in the hospital. On them lay patients who were going to have their insides taken out or something just as dramatic. Like Doll. We never saw her again. The patients cheered when she went off on the trolley and promised her a full and satisfactory sex life with her George after the stitches came out and she went home. She never did go home. Having her insides taken out did her no good at all. She had done her last bit of washing up, and giggled for the last time over George's amorous, drink-inspired advances.

Lizzy was luckier. She only had germs to fight but the fight took a long time and when it was over Lizzy was a tired old woman and no longer interested in anything her husband might have to offer her. Sepsis was a word that kept the surgeons awake at night. Often the things they used to fight it were as dangerous as the thing itself. Penicillin was less fashionable than my father's mouldy cheese. It was to be a long time before it shifted the balance of power of nursing as we knew it to one quick jab and it will all be over.

As well as the main theatre that everybody used we had our own small theatre next door to Lavender's office on the corridor. Trolleys lined up here by day and night. None of the patients on them were waiting to have their insides taken out. They were waiting to have what was left of their unwanted babies removed. This occupied a junior houseman almost full time. He sat in front of a patient scraping out bits and pieces which often included interesting little mementoes like ends of rusty knitting needles, crochet hooks, bent wire, lumps of soap and chunks of slippery elm, all of which had been used to bring about the desired result and all of which had failed lamentably to do so. The women he worked on were sometimes young and pretty. They either lived or died. Betty lived long enough to tell us why she was dying. She wasn't married and when she found out she was pregnant she told her mother who popped down the road to tell her own mother who gave them a lot of useful advice.

'You don't have to worry about a little thing like that,' she told them comfortably. 'Getting rid of it's as easy as falling off a log. Me and the woman as lived next door when I was a young wife used to get rid of each other's. We used to use crocheting hooks. A couple of days with us feet up and nobody any the wiser.' It might have been all right for granny and the woman as lived next door, but none of it worked for Betty. Not that they didn't try. They tried everything, she told us, still laughing in spite of knowing she was about to die. They tried gin and nutmeg with Betty jumping on and off a chair while granny held the cup of gin to her lips. Even we grinned at the picture that conjured up. Then granny tried the crocheting hook and that didn't work either, so finally they raked up enough money between them to go to the herbalist on Mansfield Road who had just finished one of his spells in prison and was back in business again. He took the money off them but had got so out of practice while he was in prison that the police had to be called in. They took him off to prison again and brought Betty in to us to die. She was still beautiful when she died.

Not all the unwilling mothers-to-be who found their way to our small theatre were as beautiful as Betty. Some had grown old before their time with having too many children far too quickly. They also had turned to granny or the next-door neighbour, or if they could afford it, to the herbalist, and had been sadly let down. If they were lucky enough to escape with their lives they vowed never to use a crochet hook again but go on the pill. Not the modern Pill, but the little white pills the makers claimed were worth a guinea a box. So they may have been, but it took more than a boxful of the things to shift the unwelcome little stranger that tossed and turned in its watery cradle.

We hated the herbalists with a bitter hatred. Not for the damage they did to our patients, but for the damage they did to our off-duty. When trade was brisk and they were working up to a fresh lot of porridge, Lavender had all the excuse she needed to stop our days off. I had been there almost two months before she strolled into the sluice one morning to bring me the glad tidings.

'I suppose you'd better have a day off tomorrow,' she said, looking round the enamel-ware as if seeking for a reason why I shouldn't. 'Where do you live?' I told her. Her face went ashen with anger. 'Does that mean you'll want to go home?' I said nothing. 'Well, does it?' Cornered, I nodded. 'So I suppose you'll want an evening off today and a sleeping-out pass?' She was working herself into a fury. 'You'll have to go to the Matron for a sleeping-out pass, though how I am expected to run a ward with no nurses, only she can tell me. Not that you are any good, but better than nothing I suppose.' She gave me time to digest this crumb of praise then she started again.

'Well don't just stand there, get your cuffs on and go and change your apron and tidy yourself up for the Matron.'

I stood after she had gone, weighing up the perils of a visit to the Matron against the joy of going home, then I went across to change my apron.

Not having sent for me this time the Matron was even less pleased to see me than she had been before.

'Yes?' she said unhelpfully after I had safely descended the step and avoided the dog.

'Please, Matron, may I have a sleeping-out pass?' I asked humbly. She stared at me in cold wonder.

'And what would you be wanting with a sleeping-out pass?' she demanded.

'Please, Matron, I've got a day off tomorrow and I would like to go home.'

'And where do you live?' I told her.

'And where exactly is that?' I told her. She reflected on the information for a long time before she arrived at a decision.

'You realize, Nurse, that a sleeping-out pass is a special privilege and not to be taken lightly. However, if, as you say, you intend to use it to sleep under your parents' roof I suppose you must have one.' Considering the paucity of our social life, our chances of using a sleeping-out pass for anything more exciting were extremely remote. She wrote out a pass and handed it to me. 'And see that you are in the nurses' home not a minute later than ten o'clock. Having a sleeping-out pass is not a licence to keep late hours. Tell your mother to see to it that you leave home in plenty of time to be in by ten.'

'Yes, Matron. Thank you, Matron,' I muttered effusively

and stumbled from the office with the precious piece of paper clutched in my hand.

If distance was a factor that decided whether or not we should go home on our days off, the state of our finances was of equal importance. Getting freedom forced on us at such short notice meant that we were usually unprepared for any expenses it might incur. I needed three shillings for the train fare home and this was as hard to come by as the sleeping-out pass had been. All I had was one shilling and ninepence, which left me with one and threepence to find before the evening. Pay day was a dim memory and I knew no one richer than myself who might lend me the money. Davies and the Irish girl were as broke as I was and needed the little they had left to keep their nerves going until pay day again with cheap cigarettes. I was just beginning to see my visit home fade into nothing when Davies came up with a brainwave.

'I know,' she said, 'instead of going across to dinner, go to the sitting-room instead. There will be nobody in there and you can give the chairs and sofa a good going over.' And this was what I did. I dug and came up with ninepence and bleeding fingers. I was still sixpence short.

It was while I was putting the ninepence in my purse with the rest of the money for safe keeping that I noticed the stamps my mother had sent me in despair at not getting regular letters from me. There were six penny ones. I took them back to the ward with me and waited until Lavender and the staff-nurse were safely tucked away in the office having their after-dinner cup of tea, then I hawked the stamps round the ward and found buyers for them. One woman gave me twopence for hers instead of a penny, because, as she said, it had saved her going to the post office when she got home though I suspected she had never written a letter in her life. I accepted the gift in the spirit it was given.

At six o'clock I rolled my sleeves down, put on my cuffs and knocked at Lavender's door.

'Please, Sister, may I go?' I asked.

'Go? Go where?' she said, aghast at the very idea that one of her juniors should have the nerve to want to go anywhere.

'Please, Sister, it's my day off tomorrow and I've got a sleeping-out pass.'

'Never,' she said decisively, and went back to whatever she was doing at the desk. It was not in my nature to question authority so I turned to walk out of the office. She swung round in her chair.

'Come back here at once,' she bellowed. I went back.

'Is the sluice tidy?' she asked.

'Yes, Sister,' I said.

'Are all the bathrooms tidy?'

'Yes, Sister,' I said.

'They had better be,' she said.

'Yes, Sister,' I said.

'Well what are you standing there for wasting my time, if you're going go.'

I went, trembling.

Chapter Ten

GOING HOME TURNED out to be a mixed blessing. It was one of those events where the anticipation is more pleasurable than the realization. At first anyway.

As the train neared the station and puffed past the house I was bubbling over with excitement. I could imagine the delighted astonishment as I walked so unexpectedly through the door, my father's joyous greeting, my mother's warm embrace. I should have known better. Such emotional extremes would have been entirely out of character. Nothing was as I had tried to think it would be; everything was as I should have known it would be.

Even before I got to the cart-track the excitement had died down quite a lot. It was a long way from the station and the lane had been longer and darker than I remembered it being. Night creatures howled and hooted in the trees and rustled in the hedges. Things shot across the road or sat still until I fell over them. I was glad there was a moon, but I was terrified of its shadows. I ran the last few yards with fiends chasing me and my heart pounding. Two months of urban life had spoiled me for truly rural living.

When I finally reached the door it was barred and bolted. My father always locked up early in the winter. He locked up early in the summer as well but never before eight. It was well past eight and still winter. I hammered and waited and hammered again. In the house I could hear my parents mumbling and grumbling and speculating on who could be daft enough to come knocking at that hour of the night. It was my mother who solved the mystery by drawing back the bolts and unlocking the door. In one hand she waved the hurricane lamp and in the other she brandished a poker. She peered at me and lowered the poker.

'Oh it's you,' she said huffily. 'Funny time of night for you to turn up. You'd better get inside then I can lock up again.' Deflated, I got inside.

'Look who's here, Bill,' she shouted to my father. He didn't look. He just went on smoking his pipe and staring into the fire as if he hadn't heard her.

'I suppose you'll be stopping the night,' my mother said, and seemed a bit annoyed when I said I would.

'The sheets'll be damp,' she grumbled. 'They'll have to go in front of the fire to air.' I apologized for the trouble I was putting her to by my untimely arrival and she got the bed-linen out of the bookcase cupboard behind the living-room door.

'It's my day off tomorrow,' I explained, but she was too busy crashing about with the clothes horse to pay any attention.

When the sheets and pillow cases were steaming between us and the fire, I looked round the lamp-lit room in amazement. If the lane and the cart-track had stretched during my absence everything in the house, including my mother, had shrunk. The beams in the ceiling seemed lower and the bacon and ham pictures on the walls pressed in upon me, almost suffocating me with their nearness. Disloyally I thought of the vastness of the mess-room I had left behind me.

'Are you all right there then?' my mother asked suddenly. Thinking she meant was I sitting comfortably behind the steam screen I nodded.

'Yes, thank you,' I replied politely.

'No, I mean are you all right at the hospital.' My father spat in the fire, crammed more tobacco in his pipe and settled himself back in his chair. Taking this for an invitation to talk I talked. I told them about the Matron, about Mary and about Lavender, leaving out the bits I thought they would sooner not hear. I told them about Davies and the Irish girl and the flood in the sluice. I told them little anecdotes about the patients, carefully censoring them before I told them. I was quite sure my mother had never heard of using crochet hooks for getting rid of babies, and I had no intention of enlightening her on such matters. Neither did I tell her about the Irish girl's beads; they would have shocked her as much as the abortion racket.

Though my father listened attentively he only spoke once. 'Do they feed you properly in that place, Birdie?' he asked, and I knew I had come home.

The knowledge did nothing to make the next day an outstanding success. Things I had accepted without question before I left home now stared me in the face and embarrassed me. The worst of these were the visits round the back. I longed for a door that fastened, and the pleasure of a quick read of a page of *The Farmer's Weekly* was no compensation for a lavatory chain and purpose-made toilet paper. The crowning shame was when a train went slowly past and the driver, happy to see me home again, waved to me and threw a lump of coal at me. I shrank into the corner feeling as Eve must have felt when she discovered she was naked. The driver went back to his controls looking very disappointed.

Even though it wasn't Sunday, my mother made a Yorkshire pudding for dinner in my honour. As delicately as I could I pointed out that the proper way to serve it was in a small square laid beside the meat and vegetables. 'New-fangled rubbish,' said my mother and gave me a huge wedge steeped in rich meat gravy. I ate it hungrily. I had forgotten what the real thing tasted like, but I was still glad none of my new friends were there to see me eating it.

The snobbery lasted until I was old enough and wise enough to see it as snobbery, then I went back to reading *Peg's Paper* among the nettles as happily as I had done before, though I drew a line when it came to waving to the trains.

At the end of the day I walked down the lane and back to the station with a little sadness, but not nearly as much as I had felt when I first left home.

When I reported on duty the next morning neither Lavender nor the staff-nurse greeted me warmly and asked me if I had enjoyed my day off. The moment they saw me they made a bee-line for me. Lavender got there first.

'A fat lot of good you're going to be,' she said, with her usual lack of preamble. 'First it's days off and now it's lectures. Well, you'll just have to have your lectures in your off-duty and if you don't like it you'll have to lump it. What's the use of having juniors if they're never there when you want them? Days off never should be allowed and I shall tell the Matron so when I see her in the morning.' The staff-nurse nodded in agreement and they flounced off leaving me no wiser than I was before the attack. I went down to the sluice to find out from Davies what it was all about.

'Oh, it's just Lavender going mad as usual,' she moaned miserably. 'We both start our lectures tomorrow, three a week. She's supposed to send us in ward time but when we're busy we have to have them in our off-duty.' I did a bit of rapid calculation and came to the conclusion that what with our meals being part of our off-duty and now our lectures as well, smoking time would be cut considerably unless we speeded up our eating habits. (I had by this time become part of the smoking set in the library, instead of being just an innocent bystander, which was one of the things I hadn't bothered to tell my mother.)

Our lectures were given to us by a sister-tutor who was only slightly less frightening than the Matron. Like the Matron she was high-busted and well-corseted; like the Matron she had the gift of remaining calm in the teeth of disaster. But unlike the Matron she was made of mortal stuff. She didn't only teach us, she cared for us. Our successes were hers and our failures too: not simply because they brought her credit or shame, but because she was happy for us when we passed our finals. She was a very noble woman.

It was Davies's luck to go to the lecture when she should have been working and it was me who shared my off-duty with the bread and dripping, the bed-making and the apron-changing. Both of us got to the lecture-room late, Davies because Lavender had turned funny at the last minute and refused to let her go until she had finished polishing the brass door-knobs all through the ward, and I because I had needed a quick fag to bolster me up for the experience of going back to school. Sister-tutor was also late and the lecture room was a hum of voices. Included in the class were several of the newly arrived male nurses who were passing the time away sorting out the ones they fancied on the female side. Inevitably their unanimous choice was Pickford. They were wasting their time; she was not for them.

Pickford was a very beautiful young woman. Because of her beauty she was more experienced in the ways of the world and of men than the rest of us were. She was much sought after by the members of the medical staff, particularly the older ones, so the male nurses were beneath her notice. Not that this stopped them hankering after her. All of them realized she was the best thing that would happen to them for the next three years.

The rest of us accepted her beauty and her worldly superiority over us and liked her in spite of it all. She was never reticent about her conquests and none of us grudged her them. We would sit for hours on her bedroom floor sharing the thrills of her love-life while she ate the pig's feet which, as well as men, she was inordinately fond of. She often kept us waiting in terrible suspense for the next episode while she tore a strip off a trotter and stuffed it in her mouth. We were willing to wait, knowing it would be worth waiting for.

Once a month she burst into someone's room with the news we had been waiting for with a mixture of anxiety and feline hopefulness.

'It's all right, you can stop worrying. It was a false alarm again.' And we would stop worrying but go on marvelling that yet again she had escaped retribution for her sins. It never occurred to us then to suspect that she made most of it up for our benefit, and even if we had suspected it we would have thrust the suspicions to the back of our mind. The fiction was far more exciting than the fact could ever have been. Pickford was the spice of our lives, the unattainable goal of the male nurses and a headache for the sister-tutor.

The lectures we shared with the male nurses were fraught from the start. For most of us it was the first time we had encountered the opposite sex in such numbers and having to sit in silence while our anatomical differences were brought to light was sometimes more than we could manage. Each fresh revelation was greeted with an undercurrent of suppressed giggling. Sister-tutor put up with this for some time, then after a more than usually bad time she took us in hand. She drew herself up to her full height of not an inch under six feet and in a voice of thunder she established her position.

'Nurses,' she boomed, 'I have never presumed to call myself a lady, but a gentlewoman I most certainly am. I beg that you will bear this in mind and accord me the respect that is my due,' then she sat down again. We were filled with admiration at her speech and bore her gentlewomanly qualities in mind until we almost broke blood vessels trying not to laugh. It was Pickford's fault that our memory eventually failed us. Or rather because of her.

We had been kept on the edge of our chairs trying to concentrate while sister-tutor held forth on the right and wrong method of catheterizing a male. Not a giggle was heard; the subject was too delicate even for us to laugh at.

'And finally, Nurses,' she concluded, without flinching, 'the ideal condition for catheterizing the male is to have the organ on the stretch.' There was a moment of awful silence. This was worse than anything that had gone before. We were battling with our embarrassment and struggling to maintain a decorous quiet when, from the back of the room where the male nurses sat, came a voice, loud, clear and firm.

'Send for Pickford, I presume.' There was a sharp intake of breath round the room while we waited for sister-tutor's reaction. If she lost any of her confidence she didn't show it and went on with the lecture as if nothing had been said. That was the climax of our discomfort. Nothing was ever as bad again. From that day we shared the lectures and learned about each other and were nurses instead of young men and women.

If Pickford had been making most of her adventures up for our benefit she certainly had me fooled. One morning when we were making beds together after we had been nurses for a year or two a dreamy look came over her face.

'You can't imagine the terrible thing that happened to me last night,' she said, abandoning the bed we were making while she talked. Remembering the terrible things she had boasted about in the past, nothing would have surprised me. I didn't bother asking her to tell me; she had every intention of doing so.

'Well, you remember that man I told you about, the one with the car?' A car was still the acme of affluence. 'He's not only got a car but he lives in an enormous house out at Edwinstowe and he took me there last night.' I gasped. Such daring. Such depravity. A stab of envy shot through me. Nothing like that ever happened to me. Not on such a grand scale anyway.

'You're never going to believe this,' went on Pickford. I was prepared to believe anything and so was the old man whose bed we were supposed to be making. His eyes were bulging and he was shivering slightly, but not merely because he was lying with no bedclothes on. He was as enthralled by Pickford's nocturnal adventure as I was. 'Well, when we got to this big house in Edwinstowe he took me up to a bedroom where there was a huge four-poster bed.' Pickford never did things by halves. 'He showed me a wardrobe full of fur coats and told me I could have any one I liked if I would—'

'Nurses, stop that chattering and get on with the beds,' called the sister from the door. I never did find out what the conditions were that the man attached to the coat but as I never saw Pickford wearing one I was forced to the conclusion that she had chickened out at the last minute and stood firm in the teeth of temptation. The old man died soon after, but whether from natural causes or because the excitement generated by her story was too much for him was never established. The anticlimax at the end might also have hastened his end.

Pickford's career at the hospital came to an abrupt close the night an elderly doctor, inflamed with passion for her and coldly rejected by her, waited for her on the drive with a scalpel. Their shadows were seen in dancing conflict among the rhododendron bushes and Pickford had yet another miraculous escape. Unfortunately she was made to pack her bags so fast that we never got a first-hand account of the incident. Her version of it would certainly have been more colourful than it actually was. With her romantic dreams and her pig's feet she had brought a little excitement into our lives, and our lives were pathetically short of excitement. We missed her when she went – but luckily for us, and Pickford, this was quite a bit later in our training.

At the end of three months we came off Lavender's ward with a wealth of knowledge out of all proportion to the time it had taken us to accumulate it. Much of what we had learned was more negative than positive. What not to do came easier than what to do. We had become expert at dodging issues that might have got us sent to the Matron; we had become adept at getting ourselves out of awkward situations. Never having been encouraged to think for myself I was only too happy to have someone do my thinking for me. Never having stood up for myself, except in the solitary issue of the combinations, I was easy prey for the savagery of thwarted sisters and anyone else who cared to jump on me. I was the flea that bigger fleas lie in wait for. I shrank when boldness might have served me better.

Sometimes we were unhappy but we learned to cope with our unhappiness. For most of us the discipline and restriction to our freedom was a continuation of what we had been brought up to expect. We were taught at home and at school to respect our elders and live in trembling fear of our betters. We accepted the slings and arrows of our new life as the price we had to pay if we were ever to become nurses.

But however unhappy we may have been, we stayed. Once in the profession we were committed for one reason or another. I could never have gone home anyway. My mother would have taken one look at me and my tin trunk and sent us both back to Nottingham on the next train. The dedicated ones stayed and became even more dedicated as the years went by. The middling ones stayed and were still only middling at the end of it all. Even the cruel ones stayed, and there are a few in every hospital, but they were in the minority. Most of us tried to be kind, and did our work with as much patience as we could muster. We had to on Lavender's ward. With all her ranting and raving she would have had it no other way.

Chapter Eleven

NONE OF US looked forward much to change day. If we had been reasonably comfortable for the past three months we resented being torn from our comfort. If we had been uncomfortable, there was always the chance that the devil we were about to get acquainted with could be even worse than the devil we had known and feared on our previous ward. Leaving Lavender was not the joy we had expected it to be. However harsh her justice may have been we realized it was tempered by her scrupulous impartiality; she treated all her juniors with the same wicked malevolence. What was wrong for her yesterday would be just as wrong for her tomorrow; anything which by some miracle had been right for her one day would still be right the next. We expected no lenience from her and she was never lenient; we expected no praise and were seldom praised. Like harassed salesmen our targets were constantly being raised beyond our achievements. She was angry most of the time, but when she smiled on us, we could be sure we had well and truly earned her approval just as we had earned her displeasure. A compliment from Lavender was almost worth the misery she put us through before we got it. We left her ward with a sound basic idea of what good nursing was all about: she was a yardstick to measure others against. Some matched up to her; others fell sadly below; but few improved on the standards she set, though their tempers may have been a bit sweeter.

On Sunday morning we swallowed as much of our kipper as we had time for then stampeded across to the notice board to read the change list. My heart sank. I was down for Male Medical. I had hoped for something a bit less frightening, like the Children's Block, where the sister had a reputation for sitting in her office most of the time, drinking tea with the housemen and not troubling herself too much about the running of her ward. After three months of Lavender's rigid rule I could have done with a sister like that.

Davies was having the vapours as well. She was down for Female Sanatorium which was practically out in the Styx. She was terrified.

'Will I catch TB?' she asked anxiously. I assured her that it was highly possible and she went off in a state of depression. The Irish girl was invoking the saints to preserve her. She was going to Lavender and we had told her enough about the joys of Gynae to put her off it for ever.

I reported to the sister on Male Medical and was greeted with a warmth that thoroughly confused me. I had known nothing like it before. She was fat and elderly and from the way she walked she had a lot of trouble with her arches. She bustled towards me with her arms outstretched.

'So you are to be my new probationer?' she gushed, taking my hand in hers. I struggled to get free but she only held on tighter. 'Now isn't that nice? I'm sure we are going to get on famously together.' She held me at arm's length and started having doubts. Her smile faded slightly; then, rallying, she renewed it. 'Come into the office with the others and we'll have a nice cup of tea and a little chat.' I thought of the way Lavender had greeted me and followed her into the office wondering why I felt so ill at ease. The others were standing by the desk shuffling their feet and looking just as insecure.

My new ward sister was as unlike Lavender as it was possible to be. She was nice or nasty, strict or lax, sweet or acid as the mood took her. Nobody knew from one minute to the next how they were going to find her.

A brand new young doctor with revolutionary ideas arrived at the hospital once. Like the new broom he was he tried to sweep everything clean, starting on Male Medical. On one of his rounds he stopped to examine a chronic hypochondriac who had established himself for life on one of the verandahs with a panoramic view of the surrounding countryside. At the end of an intensive search when he could find nothing wrong with the man, the doctor took out his pen and wrote across the case sheet with a flourishing scrawl, 'This man's health and temper appear to fluctuate with the weather and other considerations. We will discharge him.' The man was still there enjoying the view long after the doctor had taken his revolutionary ideas somewhere else.

The same diagnosis could have been made on my new ward sister and she was as firmly entrenched as the patient.

When we were all standing to her liking in the office she poured herself out a nice cup of tea and sat looking at us while she drank it.

'Well,' she said at last, wiping the tea off her trace of moustache, 'I can only hope you'll be a bit better than the last lot were.' Modestly we kept quiet.

'All I can say about them is that some of them are in for a shock when the Matron reads their ward report.' We sickened, trying not to think of the day three months ahead when she would undoubtedly be saying exactly the same thing about us to her next batch of nurses. She looked at me fondly.

'And as for the junior probationer, she was the worst I have ever had to put up with. I'm sure you could never be as stupid as she was.' I smirked at her and didn't know what to say which proved to her that I would be just as stupid. She lost interest in me at once.

When she had finished running down her last lot of nurses she started on the patients. Whinnying, she let us into the secrets of their disgusting habits, the demands they were likely to make on us unless we put our foot down and let them know we were not there for their convenience, and the infuriating way they had of doing all the wrong things at the wrong time. 'Why,' she said, 'somebody actually collapsed in the middle of us giving out the dinners the other day. It was most inconvenient. He just had to wait until I gave out the puddings and of course by that time he was dead. Stupid man.' She dwelt on the fallibility of human weakness for a moment or two then went on. 'And never let me see any of you giving bottles and bedpans except at the proper time. After meals is the only time I allow them to be given and if anybody wants one in between they must just wait. I won't have the patients pandered to on this ward, do you understand,' All of us except Weldon nodded in agreement. She refused to commit herself.

The sister whinnied again. She looked round us all and delivered her final warning. 'After all, if we start making them too comfortable they'll never want to go home, will they?' Again with the exception of Weldon we agreed that they wouldn't.

Abruptly she turned off the charm. She rose to her feet, swept the tea things aside and bundled us out of the office. 'Come along now, Nurses, we can't sit about all day drinking tea. I can see I'm going to have as much trouble with you as I had with the other lot if I'm not careful.' By this time none of us knew where we stood with her. We were not long finding out. After a few days she had sorted out which she liked and which she didn't. Those she liked basked in the warmth of her favouritism and could do no wrong. Those she didn't like could do nothing right for her. I was one of the unfortunates, and so was Weldon, but for a different reason. I quickly proved that I was as stupid as the former junior probationer had been, if not more so, but Weldon was a born nurse. She was kind to the patients and would have done anything in her power to see that they were happy and comfortable. None of this went down well with the sister.

'Nurse Weldon, stop pandering to that patient at once and get on with the polishing,' was a cry we heard only too often ringing down the ward. Weldon would look demure and say, 'Yes, Sister,' and carry on with whatever she was doing for the patient, in the totally mistaken idea that arranging someone's pillows so that he could breathe more easily was more important than getting on with the polishing. Doing the polishing properly would have earned her far more credits in her ward report, but it was no use trying to tell Weldon that. She had very definite ideas on a nurse's role and if they clashed with the sister's she had the courage to stand up to her convictions. The patients never properly appreciated the sacrifices she made for them. They knew which side their bread was buttered and only gave us their allegiance when the sister's back was turned. She could make things very unpleasant for them unless they kept in her good books so they sucked up to her and ingratiated themselves in order to get chicken for dinner instead of mince, and permission to smoke out of hours, both of which were grace-and-favour privileges. Weldon could give them none of these things; she only brought them and herself trouble.

I also knew which side my bread was buttered. Unlike Weldon I preferred sister's smiles to her frowns and watching the favourites in the race for her smiles I soon learned that flattery could get me a long way; if not everywhere. I crept a little and crawled a little, throwing away any scruples I may previously have had about either: for who needed scruples when one's comfort for the next three months depended on keeping the sister happy? Only born nurses like Weldon, and I had never claimed to be a born nurse.

Nothing in my experience had prepared me for being put on a men's ward so soon. Despite the few anatomy lectures we had had and Brian's elementary education in church I had still only the vaguest idea of what men looked like below the waist. I looked round the ward and saw forty men, most of them old enough to be my father, and trembled at the thought of bedpan rounds and 'doing the backs'. Surely I thought, I would never be expected to turn them over and press them to my bosom as I had done the women, while the nurse on the other side treated their rear end with her healing balm. I walked down the ward and between the two rows of men, trying not to hear their comments as I passed.

'Eeh by gum, she's a right bonny 'un,' I heard one of them say. 'Bonny' in Nottinghamshire meant fat rather than fair of face. My ego was shattered from the start. I caved in my chest, tightened up my abdominal muscles and continued my journey to the sluice.

Weldon was already warming up the bedpans when I got there but she stopped as soon as she saw me. She was as senior to me as Davies was and just as happy to pass on her position of first probationer to me. She pointed to a trolley full of bottles and bedpans.

'You'd better start giving that lot out,' she said casually. I stared at her incredulously. She looked back at me calmly with her beautiful china-blue eyes. I made a firm stand.

'What me, to all those men? I'd rather die.'

'Don't be daft,' she said, 'all you have to do is hand them whatever they want and they'll do the rest. Except for the chronics of course. They usually need a bit of a hand with theirs.' She went into no further details and with sweat oozing from my armpits I trundled the trolley into the ward. I could feel every eye on me and my face burning.

The first few beds were comparatively easy. The men accepted my offerings with a glazed look of gratitude. They had waited a long time for them. It was when I reached the cot-beds that my troubles began. I stood beside the first one with bottle held at arm's length and after a quick look turned my head away. Like the chronics on Lavender's ward the old men seemed happier when they were bare. After the one quick glance I had a clearer picture of what men looked like below the waist. I stood holding the bottle for a long time. Suddenly the methuselah in the bed took hold of my arm and started shouting at me.

'Come along, girl,' he yelled. 'Don't just stand there. Put it in, put it in.' It took a little while for it to register what I was supposed to put in and where I was supposed to put it, and when it did I got the cot rails up fast and flew back to the sluice. Weldon looked at me in mild surprise. 'Have you given them out already?' she asked me.

'No, I haven't,' I said furiously. 'You'll never guess what one of those dirty old men wanted me to do.' Weldon thought for a moment then guessed.

'Oh you mean old Mr Jones,' she said, smiling warmly. 'You don't have to worry about him. He's harmless enough. It's just that he was used to valets and things before he lost all his money. He likes ordering us about; it reminds him of old times. Just go back and stick it in for him and he'll be quite happy.'

'Which is more than I'll be,' I muttered. I went back to where Mr Jones was still lying bare, waiting for me to stick it in, and I stuck it in. I took the tender morsel of wizened flesh gingerly between my thumb and finger and gently eased it into the bottle. As I did so I remembered the boastful claims of some of the boys at the back of the school bus and laid aside yet another illusion. When the operation was completed and the cot rails safely back in place I looked round the ward and realized that none of the men had even noticed the incident. I was a nurse, I had arrived. Soon I was shoving bottles down their beds and arranging small parts with my mind detached and fixed on other things.

This detachment was even more essential on the men's wards than it had been with the women. Like the women, the men thought of us as nurses and seldom as girls young enough to be their daughters. They felt free to show us things that were kept hidden even from their wives, at least until the bedroom light was out. A sudden anguished cry would stop us in our tracks as we were rushing up the ward.

'Nurse, come quick and have a look at me whatsit. Summat's gone wrong wi' it, there's a boil or summat on it.' And we would respond to the urgency of the wounded cry and go back to inspect the whatsit. Luckily for all concerned it was usually nothing more than a pressure sore for which we had our remedies. After giving the offending organ the benefit of our attentions we would duly note the complaint in the pressure book. Then in the evening, just before we were due to go off duty, the staff-nurse or sister would appear at the ward door and, in a voice that surely must have been heard all over Nottingham, they would ask the routine question: 'Nurses, have you elevated the scrotums?' Usually we hadn't. It was a job none of us enjoyed and we always hoped that if we forgot it it would be forgotten. It never was, and once the directive had been issued we got out our trolleys and dragged our screens along, going round each patient who had complained about his whatsit, arranging his small appendages on downy cushions of cotton-wool. Our job was never made easier by the running commentaries from the men who were not eligible for the special treatment.

'By heck, some folks 'as all the luck,' they would chorus enviously.

'By gum, what I wouldn't give for a bit of cotton wool meself,' they said as we passed them with our trolleys, refusing to be inveigled by their pleas. We were always glad when the scrotums were elevated.

The drudgery on the male ward was even less divine than it had been on the women's ward. As well as the back-breaking routine of scrubbing, scouring, and polishing there was the added delight of spittoons and bottles. Not to mention ash trays. The chronics often got confused about what should be done in which container and this made the work not only harder but a good deal more unpleasant than it already was. Emptying a bottle may not be everybody's idea of a gainful occupation, but emptying a bottle that had been used as an ashtray and a spittoon as well is infinitely less appealing. Weldon and I were busily scraping the tobacco ash from the spittoons when the staff-nurse came into the sluice. She had only just passed her finals and was still almost as human as we were. She worked her knuckles to the bone as much as we did to keep on the right side of the sister.

'You'd better get into the bathroom quick,' she said to me. 'It's one of sister's bad days. Her feet are aching, she's had a row with Matron and she's on the warpath.' I thanked her for warning me and went into the bathroom. Three old men sat in there warming their hands on the radiators. They gave me stony stares when I walked in.

'Excuse me, please,' I said nervously, addressing the least belligerent-looking one. 'Would you mind moving into the other bathroom, I've got to clean this one.' He didn't answer. Nobody stirred. I said it again, even more humbly than before.

'What's the silly bitch want?' bellowed one of them, cupping his gnarled hand over his ear.

'She wants us to move,' said the belligerent-looking one I had tried to avoid.

'Tell her to mind her own bloody business,' said the deaf one firmly.

'Mind your own bloody business,' replied the other, obediently. Faced with a situation I couldn't cope with I fled again into the sluice.

'What on earth's the matter now?' asked Weldon.

'It's those men in the bathroom, I think they're going to lynch me.'

'Of course they're not, they're only the old men from the workhouse. They have to sit there to keep warm. Sister won't let them sit round the stove in the ward, she says they make the place look untidy. If you ask them nicely they'll move across into the other bathroom while you clean in there.'

'I did ask them nicely and they wouldn't budge. Will you come and ask them nicely for me?' I looked at her entreatingly. She laid down her scouring powder and wire brush and went with me into the bathroom. The old men beamed at her. They bared their toothless gums and nodded their heads respectfully.

'Would you mind moving into the other bathroom while we do this one?' she asked them calmly. Without a word each man got up and shuffled past her carrying his chair. It was then that I realized what an advantage it was to be a born nurse. Not only did their caps never slip but they got instant obedience.

Later, Weldon told me about the old men. They were tramps who had spent most of their life going from workhouse to workhouse. If they had any money on them when they booked in for the night the Master took it off them as part payment for their bed and breakfast; if they hadn't they did a few odd jobs in the gardens or in the kitchens before they were allowed to leave in the morning. They all knew about this and rather than give up the few coppers they possessed, they buried them in a field or under a hedge for safe keeping. Then, after they had sweated and slaved heaving a dustbin or two about, or dug an inch or two of ground over, they reclaimed their pennies and went on their way, unless someone had done their reclaiming for them and left them totally destitute.

When one of the regulars got ill or was too frail and old to continue his nomadic life the Master sent him up to us either to be cured and discharged or to be put in one of our cot-beds where he stayed for the rest of his life bemoaning his loss of freedom. If he was able still to use his legs he sat about in the bathroom trying to keep warm, and refusing to move for nurses like me. 'They're all right once they get used to you,' said Weldon kindly. 'It's the young ones that can be a bit awkward.' She was right, they could. They were the drop-outs of the day. They came in demanding all they could get. Being used to nothing they expected the best. There was nothing glamorous about them. Most of them had long hair, not because long hair was the fashion but because even if they had ever ventured inside a barber's shop, the barber would have taken one look at them and bundled them out again before his customers got a whiff and went off first. Not only did they smell, they were usually lousy.

One day one of them was brought in right in the middle of the doctor's round, which was against the sister's rules. She glared at the grimy young man on the trolley and her nose curled.

'Get him out of here at once,' she hissed at the porter who had brought him up. 'Can't you see we're right in the middle of the doctor's round?' The porter was an old hand and knew how to deal with people like her. He ignored her hisses and went on pushing the trolley up the ward. Just as he got to where the medical men were airing their views on one of the patients, he stopped.

'Where do you want the admission put then, Sister?' he asked in a voice loud enough to be heard by every member of the visiting squad. The senior eminence swung round, leaned in an interested manner over the trolley then drew in a sharp breath and staggered back. Eminences like him were not accustomed to meeting the patients until the patients had been properly prepared for the honour.

'Well, Sister,' he said jovially from the folds of his snowy handkerchief, 'I think that will be all for today, we seem to have seen everybody.' He was out of the door before she could remind him there was still half the ward left to be seen. Seething with anger at the abrupt termination of the doctor's round she turned on me.

'Get that man into bed at once and undress him. Then you can help Nurse Weldon to blanket bath him.' Nervously I went round the screens. The boy lying on the trolley gave me a warm grin and together we manoeuvred him into the bed.

'I've got to undress you,' I said politely. 'I hope you don't mind.' I left out the bit about bathing him; that could wait.

'Help yourself, duck,' he said cheerfully. 'You do just what that old cow told you to do, don't mind me.' I minded him dreadfully but I got on with the job praying the sister hadn't heard what he called her. Personally I felt the name was inappropriate. I liked cows. I thought they were gentle creatures, placid, and easy to get on with, none of which applied to the sister, but I still felt she might have taken offence at being called one.

The boy was only a year or two older than me but he had already put me in the category that all nurses are listed under, so he didn't seem to mind it when I peeled his clothes off. By the time I came out from behind the screens, with the bundle of rags in my arms I had learned a lot. But not enough. On the way up the ward I met Weldon coming down it with the blanket bathing trolley. She gave one look at me and screamed. 'For God's sake, just look at you. You're lousy.' I looked at me and saw I was. An army of small red insects was marching in single file down my apron. I screamed as well and dropped the bundle on the floor. The sister almost broke the golden rule that nurses must never run except in cases of fire or haemorrhage and did an Olympic-type walk to find out what was going on. She took in the lousy state of my apron at a glance.

'Really, Nurse,' she said impatiently, 'why didn't you get a bag to put those filthy clothes into. Now you will have to go across to the porter's room to be fumigated and just when the dinners are due to come up. You nurses think of nobody but yourselves.' She turned to Weldon. 'I suppose you will have to leave the blanket bathing and go across to her room and sort out a fresh lot of clothes for her. Really, what you nurses are coming to I don't know.' Bleeding with shame and flea bites I went across to the porters' room. 'You're just in time, Nurse,' said one of them when I opened the door. 'Come and have a look at this lot, I bet you've never seen anything like this before.' He was right. I looked at the pack of cards he gave me and at first I thought they were the same as the ones my mother played Patience with at home. One quick look through them and I saw they weren't. Each one had a picture on it of men and women with no clothes on doing the most extraordinary gymnastic feats with each other in some very dangerous ways. I was fascinated. I certainly hadn't ever seen anything like it before. I was just settling down to go through them again with closer attention to detail and using my powers of observation to their fullest when the head porter came in. He took the cards off me and stuffed them in his pocket. 'That's quite enough of that,' he said angrily, glaring round at the other porters. 'I suppose you're the nurse Sister rang up about? You'd better get yourself in there and strip.' One or two of the porters gave low whistles and I blushed. The head porter pushed me into a small room and handed me a bowl of disinfectant. As I gave myself a good wash down it reminded me of home and the good wash downs we used to have on the kitchen table; my mother wouldn't have cared much for the fleas. I came out of the room in the clean clothes Weldon brought over for me, scrubbed and tingling and no longer lousy. That would not be the last time I had to go to the porter's room to be fumigated: nitting may not have been a regular feature on the men's wards but other less light-hearted chases were often necessary. The crab meant more to us than a sign of the Zodiac or the delicious component of a summer salad.

Not all the patients on Male Medical were old and bad tempered, middle-aged and fatherly or even young and crabby. Some were young and lively, especially after they started to get better, and though many of them regarded us as ministering angels and untouchable some of them recognized that beneath the starch there beat a human heart. When this happened and the young man was to our liking only the dedicated nipped it too sharply in the bud. The less dedicated gave the budding a little encouragement, but very discreetly. Sister would have had us to the office like a shot if she had caught us flirting with a patient. Any flirting we did had to be done when her back was safely turned. The staff-nurse didn't matter so much; she was still young and not too dedicated and did a bit of flirting herself if something a little more stylish than the average run of patients was admitted.

My first brief but passionate encounter took place behind the bathroom door after the old men had been banished, still grumbling, to their beds. The boy who clutched me hotly to his pyjamas did so not so much because of my sex appeal but because his regular girl friend was clutching somebody else hotly while he was in hospital; and because I was nearer his own age than anyone else on the ward, except for Weldon of course, and she was obviously one of the ministering sort and untouchable. She was very cross when she came and caught us behind the bathroom door. 'If Sister finds out, she'll go mad,' she said, shooing the boy back to bed. I was past caring. When he begged me to go to the pictures with him after he went home there was no need for him to beg. I had neither been to the pictures nor out with a boy in my life and the prospect of doing both in the same evening was one I was unlikely to pass over. He never turned up. I stood about in the pouring rain outside the nurses' home gates while the lodge-man looked at me suspiciously from his window, then I turned and walked sadly up the drive. Either his regular girl friend had made her peace with him or else he didn't care much for rain.

'Serves you right,' said Weldon when I told her about it the next day. Maybe it did, but that didn't stop me from mooning miserably until Harry was admitted.

Harry was a model patient. His arrival was without incident; he was brought in at the proper time for patients to be brought in and not in the middle of the doctor's round or just when the dinners came up. He merited no black looks from the sister and no impatient 'My Gods' from us. He didn't smoke, he never asked for a bottle out of hours. He ate his boiled cod and spotted dick without complaining about their temperature and if his whatsit gave him any trouble he kept it to himself. None of us caught a glimpse of it the whole time he was in. He was exceedingly dull.

After he had been in a few days we began to notice that Weldon was giving him little attentions beyond the call of duty. As far as I was concerned she was welcome to him: until his brother came to see him one visiting day, then it dawned on me that even dull Harry might have his uses.

Eric was handsome and dashing. He wore checked plus-fours, which until then I had thought were the prerogative of the equally dashing Prince of Wales. His hair was parted down the middle and he used plenty of violet oil to keep it in place. He was the type *Peg's Paper* warned all its heroines about. He was also the type I had dreamed about ever since I smuggled my first *Peg's Paper* round the back. Whenever he turned up to visit Harry I was the first on the scene to drag a stool from under the bed for him to sit on. While he was sitting on it I flitted around doing important things to the patients on either side in order to impress him. And all I succeeded in doing was to impress Harry, much to

Weldon's annoyance. Wanting him badly herself, she viewed his interest in me with increasing displeasure. I wasn't too thrilled about it myself.

On the morning he was to be discharged he walked into the sluice where I was busy unblocking a drain. He was soberly dressed in a striped suit, a stiff white collar, a bow tie and well-polished boots. He looked every inch a gentleman. I thought of Eric's plus-fours and inwardly groaned.

'Pardon me,' he said in reverent tones. I laid down the sink plunger and assured him he was pardoned. 'I wonder if you would honour us by coming to tea on Sunday and meeting my mother and the rest of the family.' I considered the proposition for a few minutes. I wasn't in the least interested in meeting his mother but if the rest of the family included Eric I could hardly wait. I accepted the invitation and he staggered from the sluice overcome by the honour I had conferred upon him. Weldon didn't speak to me for the next few days. She saw beneath my subtlety and knew I was simply using Harry to get at Eric.

When Sunday came it was only the thought of seeing Eric that sustained me on the dreary bus ride across the town. Harry and I made polite conversation which tailed off almost before it started, then we both sat looking at the advertisements on the bus windows and tried not to look at the graffiti scrawled on the margins.

Harry had primed his mother on the right and proper way to treat visiting angels. She had opened a tin of best red salmon and there were three sorts of cake on a three-tiered silver cake stand. The crusts had been cut off the bread and Eric was nowhere to be seen. I ate the tea with one eye on the door, praying for it to open and let him in.

After we had finished off the salmon and cake and a fruit dish full of Bartlett pears we went into the front room where there was a piano with built-in candelabra on both sides and a piece of satin material let into the woodwork in the front. Harry came from a musical family. When we were all settled in the parlour he and his mother sang excerpts from Gilbert and Sullivan accompanied on the piano by the father and the young sister, playing in harmony. When they had exhausted their repertoire we all joined in and sang rousing choruses from things like *The Student Prince*. I could only do a sort of miming act; the only choruses I knew were from the nonconformist hymn-books such as 'Where is my wandering boy tonight?' We were just in the middle of a very noisy tune when Eric walked in with a girl. I was consumed with jealousy. She was treated like one of the family and was clearly expecting to become the wife of Eric. He never looked my way. When he sang his contribution, which included 'Your Tiny Hand is Frozen' he put so much passion into the words that I hated the girl friend even more. Harry took me back at ten and as far as I was concerned the affair was over. But I had reckoned without Weldon, who was a darker horse than anybody gave her credit for.

When Harry wrote, entreating me to partake of more red salmon and Gilbert and Sullivan in the parlour, it was Weldon who talked me into accepting the invitation. We had started getting a half day on alternate Sundays in addition to our other off-duty and soon tea and choruses in Harry's front room became a regular feature of my life. And of Weldon's life also, for by some means that I was never quite sure about, she managed to get herself included in the invitations. Whenever we were off together, and sometimes when we weren't, she and Harry linked hands and sang sentimental ballads with such appeal that the only dry eye in the room was mine. Even Eric squeezed a tear. Weldon possessed a sweet little piping voice and had a passion for Gilbert and Sullivan, both of which she used to worm her way into Harry's affections. By the time Eric had jilted the girl who was busily stitching her trousseau, Harry was plucking up courage to do the same to me. I made it easy for him by confessing that on the nights he left me at the lodge gates at ten, I had gone straight out over the railway embankment to meet Eric. He was so shocked that he turned to

Weldon for comfort and they went about for a long time trying to look sorry for me.

Few of our entrances or our exits escaped the notice of those whose business it was to watch over us. The ward sisters bore witness to our comings and goings on their domain; Mary kept guard over us in the home; and from his stool at the lodge gate the porter waited to pounce on us and record our departures and arrivals. Glaring at us from the heights he would demand to know our name, where we were going and when we were likely to be back. The need to identify myself at such short notice gave me a lot of trouble for the first few weeks. Being known by one name for eighteen years, then having to switch to something entirely different never came easy. Often I would keep the porter waiting so long while I sorted myself out that he would turn to whoever was having a cup of tea in the lodge with him and touch his head significantly.

'By gum, mate, we doan't 'alf get 'em. Got a right one 'ere we 'ave. Doan't even know 'er own name by the looks of things.' He little knew how close he was to the truth.

The same thing happened to me when anyone called my name on a ward or in the home. I quickly got a reputation for being deaf, daft or both. Insubordinate and insolent were other labels that were unkindly attached to me, when all I was suffering from was a mental block where my name should have been. It was a long time before I spun round spontaneously when I was bellowed at.

The interest of the gate-porter was centred not so much on our departure from the hospital as on our return to it. Deadline in the evening was ten o'clock unless we had one of the hard-to-get late passes or a sleeping-out pass. The late pass was so hard to get it was hardly worth trying for.

'Please, Matron, may I have a late pass?'

'What for, Nurse?'

'Please, Matron, I would like to go to the theatre with a friend and it doesn't finish until half past.'

'Then you must come out before the end must you not, Nurse?'

'Yes, Matron.' And no late pass.

'Please, Matron, may I have a late pass?'

'And what for, Nurse?'

'Please, Matron, I would like to go to Goose Fair.' If the nurse had said 'Please, Matron, I am going to be raped,' the Matron could not have been more shocked. Goose Fair was out of bounds; it was a hotbed of sin; it was no place for young girls to be found; it was absolutely no reason for getting a highly valuable and extremely rare late pass. Any nurse going to Goose Fair and being found out was under a shadow for a long time. We soon gave up begging for a late pass for whatever reason and accepted that officially ten o'clock was the time to book in at the gates. This had been fine while I was eating Harry's tinned salmon. Being of a blameless character he had seen to it that I was never in late. However frenzied the goings on in Heidelberg became, the Student Prince always sobered down in time for Harry to get me in by ten. But Eric was different. His night only just began where Harry's left off. I quickly realized that if I was to keep him interested the curfew was something that would have to be got round; an alternative route would have to be found into the home ground, carefully avoiding the lodge-man. In order to receive instruction on this I would need the help of a specialist and the only specialist I could think of was Pickford. We discussed my problems in the library one morning over a couple of cigarettes. She was very understanding. Though she was now a specialist she remembered the days when she also was a novice. She gave the problem her undivided attention for a few minutes.

'Have you tried bribing the lodge-man with a packet of Park Drives?' I confessed that I hadn't.

'No, well, it doesn't always work,' she admitted sadly. 'Some of them are too bloody good for this world, turning up their noses at a packet of fags.' She offered me one of her 'four for your friends' and settled down to have another think.

'We used to be able to creep under the lodge window

and run up the drive with our shoes in our hands so that the gravel didn't make a noise, then they lowered the window and got wise to it. Those bloody porters have ears like foxes, they don't miss a thing.' She walked across to the uncurtained window and stared thoughtfully through it.

'You'll have to start coming in down the railway bank,' she said at last. 'It's the only really safe way to dodge the gates.' I looked out of the window. The railway bank was a sheer drop into the nurses' home grounds and didn't seem at all safe to me. Pickford noticed my anxiety.

'You don't have to worry too much about the drop. There's a path right through it that we slither down, it gets a bit muddy in the winter, but you just have to pick out the dry bits. You do sleep on the ground floor, don't you?' I promised her I did.

'Always remember to leave your bedroom window open an inch or two when you're going to be in late then all you have to do is push it up and climb in.' I thanked her for her help, gave her one of my Park Drives and went on duty. It seemed that all my troubles were over. They were not.

What Pickford had forgotten to tell me was that the success of the venture depended on a lot of forward planning. Not only was it necessary to open the bedroom window an inch or two but it was of vital importance to see that a dustbin was placed in a strategic position beneath the window to bridge the gap between the ground and the sill. But even more important was the need to warn the other occupants of the bedroom of our late and unorthodox entry. This I failed to do the first time I slid down the railway bank after Eric had taken longer than the permitted time to say goodnight. I had got over the difficulties of the dustbin and was half in and half out of the window when the Irish girl woke up. Davies was on holiday at the time. The Irish girl was very superstitious. She had been brought up in an area where the devil and the little people were terrifying realities. The effect the saints had on either of them did nothing to loosen their grip on her imagination. When she opened her eyes and saw my two legs dangling over the windowsill in the moonlight she ran from the room screaming and clutching her beads and her statue. I could hear her shrieks ringing out all the way down the corridor. 'Jesus, Mary and Joseph and all the saints preserve us. The devil's come for us.'

I completed my journey over the sill and by the time Mary and everybody else who slept on our corridor had flocked into the room to exorcize it, I was fast asleep in bed – albeit with my clothes on – and snoring convincingly. A lot of pointed remarks were thrown in my direction but I ignored them and slumbered on, and after the exorcists had looked under the beds and in the wardrobe they all trooped off again.

Nothing could be pinned on me, except perhaps the dustbin, but Mary and the gardeners were used to finding dustbins in all the wrong places and if the purpose they had been put to was clear to all they were never used in evidence against us. Mary had to witness our sins herself before condemning us for them.

However good we eventually became at it with practice, coming in late was never achieved without some feelings of guilt, fear and even a little remorse. Every time I stood outside my bedroom window with my pure silk Bear Brand hose in my hand (at two shillings a pair they were far too dear to risk getting them laddered) I prayed earnestly for help from above.

'Dear God,' I prayed. 'If thou wilt only let me get in just this once without Mary or the night sister catching me I promise thee I will never come in late again.' Whenever a train roared past with images in the windows of law-abiding people going blamelessly home to bed I prayed again. 'Just this once Lord, and never again I promise thee.' The 'thees' and 'thous' were put in as an extra inducement to get the Lord on my side. But despite the prayers and the promises, on my next evening if I had a date with Eric I would be standing beneath my window with the same vows on my perfidious lips, and the same pair of stockings in my hand –

we could never afford more than one pair of the best stockings at a time.

The technicalities of getting into ground-floor windows were rudimentary compared to the expertise that was needed to climb any higher. This usually involved some outside assistance.

One summer evening, when two or three of us were gathered together in an upstairs room sharing Pickford's love-life and her pig's feet, a hat sailed into the open window.

'My God, it's Billy,' gasped Pickford. Billy was an inmate down at the workhouse much given to wandering about the grounds at night frightening the nurses to death. We looked through the window and saw that it wasn't Billy, it was Baker. She stood among the flower beds on the drive below imploring us to get her in. She was by no means a first offender and if she was caught the Matron was unlikely to take a lenient view at ten o'clock in the morning. It wasn't going to be easy. Baker was tall and well-covered and it would need a lot of strength to get her up. We found an umbrella and lowered a chair down to her, then we leaned out of the window, grasped her wrists and started hauling her in. It was a long time before she stood sweating and grateful on the lino. Her gratitude was premature. There was still the chair outside, ready to testify against her when someone fell over it in the morning. A dustbin in the wrong place was one thing, but a chair firmly stuck in a flower bed was definitely another. A lot of awkward questions would have to be answered before that could be explained away.

Getting in the chair was worse than hauling in Baker had been. There was less surface exposure on the chair. Since it was for her benefit we were going to all the trouble, we made her lean out of the window as far as she could with the umbrella while we hung on to her ankles. She was still fishing about with the umbrella handle when we heard the unmistakable voice of night sister. She sounded very angry.

'And what, may I ask, is the reason for this?' we heard her say from the flower beds. Poor Baker seemed lost for words. There had to be a very good reason for hanging upside down from a bedroom window at one o'clock in the morning with an umbrella in your hand. It was something that couldn't be thought up on the spur of the moment. Our first instinct was to drop her and leave her to fight her own battles, but obeying some sort of Hippocratic oath we hung on to her. Baker continued to dangle above the night sister's head.

'Get back to your room at once,' demanded the night sister furiously.

'Yes, Sister,' we heard Baker say as we slowly began to haul her up. By this time we were all slightly hysterical, and the second journey took longer even than the first had done. She had just reached the level of the window sill when night sister remembered something.

'And take the chair in with you,' she said. Down went Baker again. By this time she had lost her sense of direction altogether and swung violently about with the umbrella, missing night sister by inches and getting nowhere near the chair. It seemed hours before they were both aboard. The blood had gone to Baker's head with all that upside-down hanging and she was feeling a bit sick.

'Bloody fine mess you made of that I must say,' she said, turning on us with as much anger as she could muster in her weak condition. We accepted her insults, making allowances for the state she was in. She rubbed her puffy ankles and wrists and went off to bed.

Whether the sister thought we had all suffered enough we never knew, but we heard no more about it, which was just as well. A pretty story it would have made for the Matron's ears.

In the springtime the path that led to the front door of the nurses' home was lined with beds of fragrant wallflowers. It was only when virtue or boredom brought us in by the proper route that we were rewarded by the full impact of their evening fragrance. Ever since those halcyon days the scent of wallflowers has signified for me a purity unmatched by any lily.

When war broke out a few years later and sandbags

lay about everywhere to be stacked up and climbed on, coming in late got a lot easier, however harder other things became. But in the days when we were still praying over our dustbins, we knew nothing of wars or the rumour of wars. We knew nothing much about anything outside our own small world of bedpans and discipline, or the thwarting of discipline. We rarely read a paper; we had more interesting things to do with our pennies than squander them on such unessentials. We listened to the wireless when we had nothing else to do, but the moment anything more informative than a weather report came on we twiddled knobs to find something to make us laugh.

We knew nothing about civil wars in distant lands that were making heroes out of so many of our thinking young men, and nothing at all about the man who was already planning on making heroes of a lot more.

Fascism and Communism were only words and Jarrow with its problems was a long way away. Everywhere was a long way away. If you were English, Ireland was foreign parts, and Scotland and Wales just as remote. When a new nurse came to the hospital and proudly told us she was from Latvia and was a White Russian the more ignorant among us immediately concluded that she was not typical of her race and the others must be black, we knew nothing about black people. Black was the colour of mourning, and of our heavy duty stockings and of our necks if there had been no time to give them a proper wash for a day or two. Black people were rare, like aeroplanes, and at the sight of either mothers lifted up their children to get a better look, or dragged them away warning of the dreadful things that might happen to them if they stared. Within the cloistered confines of the lodge gates we were as ignorant as those mothers.

But if none of us could name the Prime Minister of the day we knew all there was to know about the royal family. We shared vicariously in their triumphs and disasters, we wept over their dispatches, rejoiced over their hatches and matches and thrilled to a heaving bosom over their major follies.

Unless we had a wealthy boyfriend to treat us we could only afford to go to the pictures while pay day was still hot in our purses but at the first hint of a royal occasion we begged, borrowed or stole the wherewithal to get Pathé Gazette's version of the affair and snivelled and sighed our way through it, resolving as we wept to live a better and more useful life in future to match the perfection we were watching.

As well as having us all going about in the same shade of green and wearing little round hats with veils arranged coquettishly over one eye, Princess Marina filled us with tearful envy when she so beautifully married the dashing Prince George. I was on night duty nearly two years later when his father died. The patients on the ward refused to lie down and go to sleep; instead they sat with their earphones clamped on listening to Stewart Hibberd telling us that the King's life was drawing peacefully to a close.

I was on night duty again when the Prince of Wales, after thrilling us with his accession to the throne, renounced it. We sat dewy eyed and gasping round the wireless set that crackled and faded in the concert room. Great hissing of pent-up breath greeted the announcement that he was giving up the throne for a woman. There was not one of us that wouldn't have changed places with Wallis, however unpopular she was with the Establishment.

I left the Male Medical ward a good deal wiser and a good deal less innocent than I was when I went on it. I had learned all about creeping and crawling. I knew more about men than the average girl of the day knew when she walked spotless to the altar. My education had progressed in leaps and bounds. A Spanish friend returning home after a visit to England wrote to me. His English was not perfect: 'My wife she suffers much from the dump of London but I, from the Children's Newspaper did learn many curious and wonderful things. These being the amazing adventures of Marco Polo, how to ride a bicycle in three easy lessons and the astonishing behaviour of the ape.' I knew exactly what he meant. I too had learned many curious and wonderful things, not the least being the astonishing behaviour of the human male.

Chapter Twelve

FOR MOST OF us the first Christmas we spent in hospital was a happy time. Though many of us were far from our homes we were too caught up in the excitement of it all to gloom over the separation from our families. The excitement spread through the hospital like a virus infection. It had started as far back as October, immediately after Goose Fair week, when we began making watery cups of tea and selling them to the visitors at a penny a cup, the funds to be used for buying paper chains to decorate the ward and small gifts to give to the patients.

The money came in slowly. In sharp contrast to the shocks and thrills of the men's wards I was now on Female Chronic and the grannies got no more visitors than the poor old chronics got on any other ward. Those who did come looked the other way when we approached them with our clanking tea-urns, or smiled awkwardly and made excuses.

'Not just now, thank you, me duck. We had a cup

with us dinners before we came out, we couldn't drink another drop if we tried.' Later, when we started giving them a cup for nothing they accepted it gratefully and drank it thirstily with no thought of the one they'd had with their dinners. Pennies were not so easily come by that they could be tossed lightly into our holly-decorated collecting boxes. Most of them had already had to pay a penny or even twopence on bus fares which set them back considerably for the rest of the week.

Neither the tea nor the visitors mattered much to the patients. Many of them were too busy taking off their nightdresses and stripping their beds to notice what was going on around them. From the day they were admitted and put into a cot-bed, to the day they died still in the same cot-bed, they had to find their own amusement. Hanging their washing over the rails to dry was as good a way as any of filling the empty hours until they were discharged to the mortuary. The only time they showed any enthusiasm was when a friend or relative long since dead dropped in to have a chat with them. We were never privileged to hear the other side of the conversation but we heard enough from our own side to give us a fair idea of the identity of the ethereal visitor. While dutiful sons and daughters sat ignored by the bedside, their aged parent would be happily chatting to her own mother who, if she had lived, would be a hundred and twenty come Michaelmas. There were others who dropped in occasionally for a fleeting visit. The warmth of their welcome varied with their relationship to the patient.

'Eeh by gum, our Georgie, who ever would 'a thought of seeing you here?' a delighted mother would say, greeting a son lost without trace among the poppies of Flanders. 'By, tha's grown a big lad sin' I saw thee last. Tha gets more like thee faither every day.' And whatever the saucy boy of her memory said in answer would be wrong for her. 'Shurrup, yer cheeky bugger, or Is'll get thee dad to gi' you't strap when he comes in from't pit. He'll larn you to coss at me.' Then, grumbling and scolding, the mother would fall back on her pillows leaving Georgie to slip away as quietly as he had come.

Sometimes it was a husband who turned up to revive old memories. He usually got short shrift. Whatever he offered was spurned without hesitation.

'You can keep away from me, yer mucky sod. That's all you ever think on. I'm having nowt like that after a busy wash-day.' And the husband, rejected in death as he had so often been in life, slunk away to try his luck with the harpies in the sky, while his wife snuggled down, happy to be rid of him again.

When they were not exchanging greetings with the dead or stripping themselves and their beds bare there was nothing for the chronics to do but lie looking at nothing and seeing nothing. We fed them, bathed them, changed them and scoured their bottoms, knowing it was all done to no purpose, unless you could call the satisfaction some of us got in making them comfortable an end in itself. A contented sigh from one of them could make us feel rewarded.

The bright young doctor with the revolutionary ideas suggested one day that we should try getting some of the grannies up and sitting them in chairs. We were horrified. Our work was heavy enough already without making it heavier by tugging and pulling unwilling old ladies in and out of bed. The sister quickly scotched that idea, much to our relief. The thought of forty or fifty grannies cluttering up the ward was no more appealing to her than it was to us.

Then the bright young doctor had an even more revolutionary idea. 'Let's send some of them home,' he said enthusiastically. He stopped by Alice's cot one day and surveyed her twenty stones of wobbling flesh that took four of us to hoist on a bedpan until we gave up and let her wet her bed instead. When he had finished looking at her, he got her case-sheet out and wrote, 'This lady lies all day in bed like the cows in the fields. She does nothing, she says nothing, but she eats plenty. Send her home.' Poor Alice with her swinging breasts each weighing half a stone took such fright that she had one of her funny turns and established her right to lie in bed for the next year or two.

But where did the young doctor think home was? Like most of our grannies, and granddads too, Alice was in the only home she had known for years. Many of them had been abandoned long ago by their families who had been relieved to see them go off in the ambulance to the infirmary. It was more respectable than having them put in the workhouse and caused less talk among the neighbours. For a few weeks one or other of them would turn up with an egg or a tin of mint humbugs but after a while they lost interest and were never seen again until they were summoned to collect the death certificate. Even that caused problems. If they had been notified a little prematurely and there was still breath left in the father or mother they had been sent for to accept responsibility, they sometimes asked, a little hesitantly, to be allowed to take the death certificate away with them then, rather than have to come back for it at some inconvenient time when the kiddies were clamouring for their dinners. The sister on Female Chronic was gentle and kind, and though she frowned on the request and never granted it, she was never too hard on them for asking. She knew enough about poverty to understand that sitting waiting at a bed while its occupant took a protracted leave of it could be a costly waste of time, what with the funeral to pay f the black, and the bit of ham the rest of the mourners would expect after it was all over. Not many of them needed to be told to go home and wait and we would get in touch with them as soon as something more definite had established itself, which meant that the old ladies had to get on and do their dying alone unless one of us had time to pop round the screens now and again to see how they were getting on with it. They got on with it in much the same way as they had got on with things all their lives.

Our gallant sister-tutor, who was already dying and knew it though none of us did, put the case for the elderly in a nutshell one day when she was lecturing us on caring for the elderly.

'It is often thought,' she said with a twinkle in her eye, 'that the old become what they are through age. In my opinion this is not so. The old are as they have always been but a little more so.' She was proved right more often than not.

Old Granny Wilks was typical of sister-tutor's theory. She died as she had lived, obstreperous and independent to the last. She was the terror of the ward. Her husband had escaped early from her iron rule and left her with nothing but her fierce pride to sustain her. It never let her down.

As might have been expected she chose an awkward time – right in the middle of giving out the dinners – to start doing her dying. When somebody remarked that Granny Wilks wasn't complaining about her mince as loudly as she usually did the sister sent someone across to find out why. The nurse took one look at Granny Wilks and hurried as fast as the law allowed to fetch the screens. She was busily arranging them round the bed when Mrs Wilks opened one eye, took in the screens and the nurse's reverent hush and reacted sharply to both.

'I isn't dead yet, my lass, nor isn't likely to be this side of teatime, so you can put them things back where you got them from and look sharp about it. I'll go when I'm ready and not a minute sooner.' Then she settled herself back on her pillows and went when she was ready, which was right in the middle of giving out the teas, thereby causing a great deal of inconvenience which would have suited her fine.

Gwenny was different. Gwenny had never dealt with a crisis single-handed in her life and certainly wouldn't have known how to cope with dying alone. She had three sons and a daughter. When the daughter was born Gwenny had looked down at the infant, noted its sex and sighed contentedly. 'And now I can move into the spare room and be permanently too tired for Jack. I have a baby doll to dress in pretty clothes, a faithful companion for my middle years and a devoted nurse for my old age.' And so she had. Sh made it her business to see that she had. Any suitors for her daughter's hand that came knocking at the door were given tea and sympathy and sent away convinced that it would be the worst thing they could ever do to marry the daughter.

When Gwenny lay dying, the girl who had sacrificed her life to keep her mother happy came in every evening from work and stayed until it was time to go to work again. When a nurse went behind the screens one night and found her fast asleep in her dead mother's arms we wondered what cross she would take up to replace the one she had lost.

Baker, the girl we had hoisted into the bedroom window, was with me on Female Chronic. However clumsy she may have been at getting in late she was marvellous with the patients, though her methods may not have suited everybody. She would stand over them, her brown eyes soft with compassion, and bawl things at them which would have made interesting reading in the Sunday papers.

'For God's sake, if you've got to die don't do it while I'm on duty. I've got enough to do without hanging about waiting for you to die.' And somehow through the haze of her semi-conscious state, the patient would recognize the voice of authority and rally enough to take the drop of egg and milk generously laced with brandy that Baker was lovingly offering her.

The patient who had driven the rest of us mad with her unreasonable demands would get all she wanted from Baker, but with a running commentary thrown in. 'My God,' she would yell, picking up a handkerchief for the twentieth time, 'it was a bad day for us nurses when they stopped us hitting you.' And the patient would smile happily, knowing she had somehow won approval.

It was while Baker was standing beside a bed one day, gently smoothing the thin white hair of one of the grannies and hurling abuse in her ear, that Dr Collins stood for a moment at the ward door, watching and listening, and fell in love with Baker. He was Irish and had curly hair and there wasn't a probationer that hadn't suffered unrequited love for him at some time or another. He waited until Baker had passed her finals before he did anything decisive about her, but from that day she was a little less abrasive, swore a little less and never again needed to be hauled into her bedroom window. Dr Collins knew better ways than that of getting her in late.

Brooker was another nurse with us on Female Chronic. She was a third-year nurse, almost due to sit her finals. She was a quiet girl who treated us and the patients with the same reserved consideration. The stir she was to cause around the hospital was something none of us could have anticipated.

Not many of the patients on Female Chronic enjoyed Christmas as much as we did; though we did our best to include them in the festivities, the season of goodwill had long since lost its meaning for them. They ate their minced turkey with the same indifference as they ate their minced shin of beef on other days. We put up streamers and holly and blobs of cotton wool snow and did it all with a special sort of Christmassy help from the male nurses who popped in now and again to see how we were getting on with it and to hold the steps for us while we clambered up them. They never did the clambering up, they only did the jobs that suited them and it suited them fine to stand at the foot of the steps looking up our dresses.

We hung bits of mistletoe in places where they could be seen, and we hoped taken advantage of, by the junior members of the medical staff. The boy scouts brought in the tree and we decorated it with glittering stars and winged angels. We filled our old black stockings that had gone past mending with tiny tablets of soap, face flannels and cheap tins of talc that sister had been out and bought from Woolworth's with the tea money. The patients were not particularly impressed by the gifts but the giving made us feel good and added to the spirit of Christmas. We loved it. It was different from anything we had known before. Especially me.

Christmas at home had been much the same as any other time, except for the remains of the pig lying about, the plum pudding and the fowl we had for Christmas Day dinner. My father didn't like the fowl. 'Do we have to have fowl?' he asked every year. 'I don't like the bones in a fowl,' pleaded my father, in a last desperate stand.

'Then you'll have to leave them,' returned my mother helpfully. Once the pudding and the fowl had been eaten there was nothing left of Christmas except a tangerine in the middle of the afternoon and a mince pie and a tin of fruit for tea. The tin of fruit was a mixed blessing. Getting it open always meant a frantic search for the small rusty tin-opener which was never where it had been put the last time it was used. Luckily we didn't eat much that came out of a tin; my mother's temper got very frayed while she was looking for the tin-opener.

But Christmas in hospital was a time of gaiety and friendliness, with some relaxing of the rules we had to abide by during the rest of the year. On Christmas Eve we sang our carols, going from ward to ward with candles flickering in jam jars, and our cloaks turned inside out to reveal the bright scarlet linings. We cuddled the children who for various reasons, most of them sad, had not gone home for Christmas. A frantic young mother left one on our doorstep once as a special gift. We loved him dearly and called him Noel of course, though he didn't live long enough to need a name.

We kissed the more respectable-looking old men, and some of the young ones too if they looked as if they wanted us to kiss them, and all beneath our sprigs of mistletoe, which made the kissing legal. The old men liked it and begged for more. It had been a long time for them since the Christmas before. It was sometimes necessary for us to be firm about their more lecherous suggestions. We were also firm with hands that strayed across our bottoms.

When the first rush of work had been done on Christmas morning the sister took us into her office and distributed the presents and gave us cups of coffee with a dash of weak brandy from the emergency cupboard if we had a taste for it. Being strictly teetotal, I drank mine minus the brandy. It was very strong and very nasty. Coffee was not a thing we were used to drinking; coffee was for our seniors and the rich. It hadn't spread to the common herd.

The gifts that we enthused rapturously over were usually very small bottles of scent, the most popular being Californian Poppy and Nuits d'Amour, unless someone had been grossly extravagant and lashed out on Soir de Paris which put the giver and the recipient in a different class from the rest. Our popularity could be measured by the strength of our emanations during Christmas and for as long as the scent lasted after Christmas.

The sister looked suitably delighted with the Wedgwood ashtray we gave her to match the Wedgwood trinket box her nurses gave her the previous year. A lot of cigarettes had to be sacrificed to raise enough money to buy these collector's items. They were chosen with care and given with envy.

Although Weldon was not on my ward she gave me a walnut box full of luxurious writing paper and envelopes which must have cost her every penny of half-a-crown. The box was solid and had a patina which was to last my lifetime. Not expecting anything from her, I had bought her nothing so I had to rush across to my room to find something that would pass as a Christmas present. All I had was the very last pair of black woollen stockings my mother had packed me off with. I bundled them in a bit of brown paper and presented them to Weldon when we exchanged visits to each other's wards to admire the decorations. She didn't seem terribly excited with the gift. They certainly wouldn't last as long as her beautiful walnut box, though they cost just as much.

While we drank the sister's coffee we offered each other different and more exotic brands of cigarettes, with no 'four for your friends' stuck down the side. Du

Mauriers in pretty pink boxes were flourished in return for de Reszke Minors – if there was a major member of the family none of us had ever met it; the Minors were as much as we could afford. When we were all mellow with goodwill and coffee someone would produce a flat Russian sort of cigarette which made us feel very daring and often very sick.

On Christmas Day we dined in the evening like the gentry did. If we were unlucky enough to be sent across to the mess-room for a midday meal all we got was cold meat and beetroot and a lot of black looks from the domestic staff. They were far too busy with their own celebrations at that time of day to want to be bothered with us. But only the most dreary of the sisters did this; the others let us flout the rules about eating on the ward and we stuffed ourselves with nuts and dates and chocolates while we did bedpan rounds and changed dirty sheets. We stuffed the patients as well, which accounted for the extra dirty sheets that had to be sluiced and counted before the porters came for them.

We were given no official off-duty at Christmas nor ever wanted any. The morning flew by while we got the ward ready for the Mayor and Corporation to come and carve the turkey. We put clean nightdresses on the grannies and tied their hair back in skinny little pigtails with bandage bows. We put their teeth in so that smiles would look more like smiles and less like empty tombs and at the last minute we rushed round covering everything up again so that the Mayor wouldn't see anything he shouldn't. 'Who do he think he is?' grumbled the old ladies when we explained to them why we wanted them to keep covered up. 'He's no better than what we are. Got the same as us, hasn't he?' We doubted it and hoped not but didn't argue; after all it was Christmas.

When the turkey had been cut up ready for us to mince, the civic party did a round of the ward trying to keep their eyes to themselves; in spite of our last-minute efforts there were still plenty of naked ladies lying about. The naked ladies were not too interested in the civic party either. They had no idea who they were being asked to shake hands with and got them all mixed up with people they had known in the past and either screamed abuse at them, or wrung them warmly by the hand and tried to smother them with kisses, to the discomfiture of the visiting side.

'Good afternoon,' said the Mayoress to Rosie. Rosie beamed at her in instant recognition. Encouraged, the Mayoress held out her hand. Rosie grasped it and held on to it while she dived down the bed to find an offering suitable for giving to such a gracious lady. When the woman saw what it was that was being pressed into her hand she nearly fainted and the civic party rushed off in a great hurry to find a wash-room.

'You shouldn't have done that to the lady,' bawled Baker to Rosie. 'She was very cross with you.' Rosie scraped most of the gift off the counterpane and threw it on the floor.

'Them folks is all the same,' she fumed. 'Serve the stuck-up bitch right if she gets nowt else for Christmas.' Then she went back to her own world of fantasy where she was happier to be and where folks weren't as ready to spurn her gifts.

Our dinner was served in two sittings in a mess-room that had been garlanded out of all recognition for the occasion. We all preferred to go to the first sitting while the food was still hot and reasonably abundant. But whichever meal we found ourselves at, the Matron graced the head of the table in order to prove that there was no favouritism between the two sittings. She lit the fire on the puddings, usually unsuccessfully, while she successfully damped the fire of our Christmas spirit. We pulled our crackers and wore our funny hats acutely conscious of her watching us. We were not used to doing anything as mundane as eating in front of the Matron.

When the dinners were over it was time for the concert to begin. Like the socials in the village hall the concert was an annual event that took a lot of preparing for. It was presented by the more extrovert members of the medical staff, the male nurses and anyone else talented enough or uninhibited enough to offer themselves up for sacrifice. Skeleton staffs were left on the ward and as many of the patients as could make the journey were taken to the concert room. Wheelchairs, beds, trolleys and stretchers jostled each other in the corridors. Greetings were exchanged and rude comments passed. Friends and relatives came from as far afield as their feet, their bicycles or the limited bus service would carry them. Everywhere was a buzz of excitement. The exodus from ward to concert room was as much fun as the concert itself. Or almost.

By the time the entertainment began, after several false starts due to missing props, whispering loudspeakers and curtains that refused to part company, the audience was already in a receptive mood and needed no warming up to ensure the success of the evening. The programme consisted of several short but meaty sketches with a medical flavour, some parodies on the pop songs of the day in which the idiosyncrasies of the more senior staff were brought to light and immediately recognized, and a few straight acts which were never as straight as they were intended to be, the audience saw to that. Each item was rewarded with thunderous applause and enough barracking to put the artistes off the stage for ever, unless they had hides like leather. It was only when the Matron sailed on the stage that an uneasy silence descended on the audience. She obliged with a turn every year. No concert would have been complete without her.

Her magnificence was shrouded from neck to ankles in shimmering grey satin. Her hair was carved out in waves of strictest geometric symmetry and the whale-bones in her corsets were clearly silhouetted in the unflattering footlights. Her pince-nez hung from her neck on a piece of velvet ribbon.

She stood for a moment or two on the platform while she composed herself ready to go into action, her fingers loosely entwined across her noble abdomen. Those who were new to the concerts instinctively covered their ears, certain that a lady of such prima-donna proportions would have a voice to match. This was not so. After the senior registrar who was given the honour of accompanying her on the piano had run through the preliminary trills and arpeggios, she formed her mouth into a small circle, and in a voice that could be heard no further than the first three rows of chairs she gave us 'Little Brown Bird'. Because of the poor acoustics of the concert hall it took the audience a little while to realize when the song had finished, so in the best tradition of Covent Garden the applause was delayed long enough to suggest a stunned appreciation of the treat they had been given. Finally someone timidly started the clap-ping off, but it never reached the volume the other acts had produced. The Matron acknowledged the acclaim with a crackling bow, glided off the stage, and the concert was over.

Christmas was over as well as far as organized celebratings were concerned but in the nurses' home it went on far into the night. Once a year authority turned a blind eye and a deaf ear, the comings and goings from the doctors' quarters, banned at all other times, were ignored, and the sound of merrymaking, that had taken more than the lemonade in the mess-room to stimulate, kept the non-merrymakers awake and angry. The Irish girl went off with her bottle to add her contribution to the noise. Davies and I locked the door behind her and tried not to imagine the orgy that was undoubtedly going on outside it. Being teetotal was very restricting.

It was a long time before the Irish girl hammered on the door and demanded to be let in. She came in waving her empty bottle about and seemed in a happy mood but Davies and I were not. We refused to listen to her account of the party and she gave her beads a quick going over and went to bed. In the morning none of us said much. The Irish girl was going about with her head in her hands and snapped at us whenever we spoke, so we thought it best to keep our mouths shut. The atmosphere was much the same in the mess-room, with the merrymakers irritable and the non-merrymakers trying to efface themselves.

After that things got back to normal, the decorations were taken down, the trees burnt and the black woollen stockings retrieved for a bit more wear. On the change day after Christmas, Davies and I, Weldon, Baker and the Irish girl were all put on night duty.

Chapter Thirteen

Though we had expected to be put on night duty the shock of actually seeing our names on the change list in the night-duty column stunned us for a moment. We looked at each other without speaking. We had heard enough about the horrors of night duty to put us off it for ever: a night off a month if we were lucky, lukewarm mince and rice pudding for our midnight meal and again when we came off in the morning, and a night sister with a reputation as bad as Lavender's. We groaned at the prospect. Pickford was the first to speak. She was the one likely to suffer most from the upheaval. 'My God,' she wailed, looking round at us for sympathy, 'bloody nights, and I've got a date on Tuesday.' None of us answered her, we were all too concerned with our own troubles to be bothered with hers. Baker was speechless. Dr Collins only did rounds at night when there was an emergency. She needn't have worried, there were ways and means and he wasn't slow in finding them. Many a patient was to wake from a deep sleep while the nurse in charge was at her midnight meal, to find Dr Collins and Nurse Baker leaning solicitously over the bed holding hands.

Weldon wasn't happy about the move either. She and Harry had reached the stage where a semi in West Bridgford, with a piano in the parlour and plenty of Gilbert and Sullivan sheet music, was a foregone conclusion. Night duty would hamper their courtship even more than it had been hampered before.

Davies and I and the Irish girl were beset by no such problems, the Irish girl because she was still poor and saving herself to be a bride of Christ, Davies because she was still too shy to say 'Yes' when one of the male nurses asked her to go to the pictures with him, and I because Eric had cast me off as lightly as he had cast off a dozen girls before me. This put me in a difficult position with Weldon. It meant that I could no longer go to Harry's with her on our Sunday off. I went once and it was so embarrassing that I left straight after tea and walked back to the hospital by myself. Nobody had warned me that Eric would be sitting there with his latest girl friend. We eyed each other up and down – possession being nine points of the law she won, and thoroughly enjoyed the afternoon. Eric at least had the grace to look a bit uncomfortable. I often wished afterwards that I had hung on to Harry instead of giving him to Weldon. A semi in West Bridgford might not have been so bad after all, and I might even have grown to like Gilbert and Sullivan.

Obeying the sister's instructions after breakfast, Baker and I went back to Female Chronic and worked there as hard as ever until second dinner, then we carted all our worldly possessions across to the night nurses' corridor and went to bed. But not to sleep, Nelly saw to that.

Nelly was the housemaid who cleaned the night nurses' corridors. She was hard-working and conscientious. She waited until she could be reasonably sure that all the night nurses were asleep then she crashed about with her buckets and mops, scrubbing floors, cleaning paintwork and washing down walls with tremendous energy. She was a happy soul until someone stepped on one of her nice clean floors, then she cursed and screamed loud enough to wake everybody on the corridor, if her singing hadn't wakened them up already. For while she worked she sang. Not loudly, or even tunefully, but with a doleful monotony that was as disturbing as her clanking buckets or the upper register of her quarrels. She only ever sang two songs. One was 'Red Sails in the Sunset', and the other 'I'm Dancing with Tears in my Eyes, 'Cos the Girl in my Arms isn't You', and Nelly sang them often. Our eyes were just getting heavy when she burst into the room.

'Come on you lot, time to get up. You'd better get a move on an' all, its nearly eight o'clock and break-fast's at half past.' She whirled out of the room. It took me a second or two to work out what she had been talking about. In my fuzzy state I distinctly remembered eating one breakfast already that day. Why I should be expected to have another was some-thing I couldn't immediately explain to myself. I looked across at the other two and saw they were as confused as I was.

'What's she yapping about?' said Baker from the bed next to mine.

'We've got to get up to go on nights,' said Strickland from the other bed. She got up and started to put her clothes back on again. She was a small pretty girl with pale fluffy hair: none of us knew much about her. The reason we knew nothing much about her was because we never got the chance to. She was never in the library or in the sitting-room. She went to the same lecture class as us but seldom spoke to anybody. Those who had worked with her seemed to know as little about her as we did. As my mother would have said, she kept herself to herself. The only friend she had was Brooker, the third-year nurse Baker and I had been with on Female Chronic. She also kept herself to herself, but there the resemblance ended. Where Strickland was soft and timid, Brooker was brisk and had an air of authority. None of us could understand what they could possibly have in common to make them so pally. We understood less the day Nelly rushed out of a room screaming and we rushed in and found Strickland lying across the bed with the bottle of Lysol still dripping on the floor. We racked our brains for reasons but the only one we could think of was that she must have been upset when Matron, inexplicably to us, sent Brooker away to finish her training somewhere else. Not that that seemed an adequate reason for killing yourself.

'Bloody stupid,' said Pickford. 'Nobody gets that stuck on a girl – except a boy of course.' Well, Strickland had, and the reason for it remained a mystery to us all for a long time.

Baker and I stayed in bed while Strickland got herself ready, then we staggered blearily round the room, dressed ourselves and went across to the mess-room. The second breakfast was the same as the first one had been, except that the kippers were warmed-up editions and tasted no better for it. We ate them then queued up at the hatch for our night nurses' baskets. These were the nicest things about night duty. They were made of wicker and had two lids and a handle. Inside each was a cup and saucer, a plate, some cutlery, a pat of butter and a freshly baked cob loaf hot from the hospital bakery. The loaf was intended to be eaten at four o'clock in the morning in the ward kitchen as a sort of afternoon tea. It had usually disappeared in buttery hunks long before that.

When we had got our baskets we queued up again at the sister's table to be told which ward we were to go on. The night sister looked me up and down. She registered my spotty chin, my sliding cap and my crooked seams and she raised her eyes to heaven. After she had recovered somewhat she consulted the roster in front of her.

'Male One and Male Two,' she barked. 'Runner.' I picked up my basket and crept away. Outside the messroom I collided with Pickford. She was to be a runner as well.

'What is it?' I asked her.

'Lowest form of life,' she answered.

'What do we have to do?'

'Everything.'

'Yes, but what?'

'Everything the bloody seniors don't do, and all at top speed. We don't get called runners for nothing.' She went off, her shoulders bowed with care. I followed her.

On Male One the nurse in charge greeted me coldly. She knew me from day duty and wasn't overjoyed at seeing me. 'Oh, it's you,' she said, disappointed. 'I hoped I might get somebody a bit decent, I wasn't expecting you.' I swallowed the insult and waited for her to get over her disappointment. 'Well, I suppose you'll have to do. You'd better go and report to Male Two then come straight back here, I'm busier than she is.'

The nurse in charge of Male Two looked at me as if unable to believe her bad luck. 'What have they sent you for?' she demanded. I apologized and said I didn't know. 'You'd better stay here now you're here, this ward's busier than Male One.' Mute with terror I stayed. Night duty was going to be even worse than they had said it was.

'Don't just stand there,' went on the nurse in charge. 'Get your cuffs off, your sleeves rolled, up and start giving out the bottles.' She walked away, then she came back and thrust a large sheet of foolscap paper in my hands. 'You'd better have a look at the duty list before you start.' I looked at the paper. On it was a fully comprehensive list of things I would be expected to do before I went off duty in the morning. I started reading it.

'Nine o'clock, report on duty,' which I had – twice. 'Nine five, go into ward,' which I hadn't. 'Nine ten, start bottle round; nine twenty, finish bottle round; nine twenty-five, go into kitchen; nine twenty-six, fill kettles; nine twenty-seven, place kettles on gas ...' At that moment the nurse from Male One came to find me.

'I thought I told you to come straight back to me after you had reported on this ward.'

'Yes, Nurse.'

'Then why didn't you come back straight to me?' I apologized and followed her back to Male One. She handed me a fresh sheet of foolscap paper. Skipping the first twenty-seven minutes I read on.

'Nine twenty-eight, mash tea; nine twenty-nine, mix Horlicks; nine thirty, make Ovaltine.' At 'nine thirty-one, give out drinks', the nurse from Male Two arrived. I cowered behind the kitchen table.

'What do you think you're doing here? Get back to my ward at once and start giving out the bottles.' I went, shutting my ears to the battle that raged in the corridor between my seniors. Whatever truce they made did not last long. Never once, during the whole of that first night was I in the place I was expected to be.

When they had sorted things out between them I gave out bottles, collected in bottles, filled kettles, lit gases, mixed Horlicks, mashed tea, made Ovaltine and wearily dragged the drinks trolleys round the wards. Most of the men got something entirely different from what they had asked for. Some accepted my mistakes and made allowances for my first night, but others were not so obliging.

'Ayupp, what dos't think this is then?' asked one of them, waving a cup of warm milk menacingly at me. 'I axed for a sup o' tea, not bloody bairn's pap.' I apologized and made the exchange. He was one of the lucky ones. By the time I got to the other ward I was throwing the wrong things at everybody and not stopping to apologize, let alone do a swap.

While I was peddling my wares the senior nurses were rushing up and down the wards attending to the vital necessities. They woke up those who were already sleeping and gave them things to make them sleep. They shook and pummelled pillows so furiously that patients who had already shaken and pummelled their own were obliged to do them again to get them where they wanted them. Noisy chronics were given injections that would make them even noisier when the effect wore off. Small aches and pains were fiercely rubbed with oils that would scent the ward and the nurse's hands for the rest of the night. Dressings were changed, tubes taken out, cleaned and put back again, poultices were rushed from the kitchen to the bedside between two dinner plates, so that the bread, linseed or mustard they were made of would still be hot enough to make the patient jump with shock when they were slapped on his back or front. The poorly ones were tepid sponged, towel dried, methylated spirited and talcum powdered until they were mighty glad when the nursing stopped. Enemas were given, temperatures taken, scrotums elevated and whatsits sympathetically examined. Not a bone was left unturned. And when it was all done the main lights were dimmed, little green cloths were pinned round the lamps above the patients who needed special care and above the table where the nurse in charge would sit to do her books and keep an eye on the sleeping patients, and we the runners were already tired and longing for our beds. With more than eight hours still to go our night had hardly begun.

When the last green cloth had been pinned in place and most of the men were asleep in spite of our attentions, the seniors gathered in small groups in the kitchen to drink tea and run down their runners, while we emerged from the obscurity of our sluices to sit in semi-limelight at the table in the middle of the ward. This carried tremendous responsibility with it. Not only were we there to keep an eye on the patients, but it was our duty to watch out for the night sister and get to the kitchen with a warning cry before she did. To do this properly required sharp eyes and sharp ears. Night sister always wore plimsolls when she did her round which made her visit harder to anticipate. She could be right on top of us before we knew she was about. Sometimes it was a patient who was the first to hear her.

'Ayupp, lass,' a sleepy voice would say in an urgent stage whisper. 'Tha'd better watch out, t'bloody night sister's upstairs, yon's her plimsolls squeaking.' And sure enough from the ward above would come the sneaky squelchy sound of rubber soles on wooden floor boards. There was a peculiar ghostly quality about the footsteps that had me racing to the kitchen the first time I heard it, shaking and sweating and wishing I had as many charms as the Irish nurse had for warding off evil spirits.

'Come quick, Nurse,' I yelled, breaking up the tea-party. 'There's a ghost somewhere, I can hear its feet.' By the time the ghost had materialized into night sister we were all in our proper places and the tea-cups out of sight.

Male Two had its own special built-in night-sister alarm. His name was Dummy. He was tall and gaunt and looked as wild as a scarecrow. His long tangled black hair stood out like wire and his eyes sank like two stones into the back of his head. He wore a striped nightshirt that flapped round his ankles and he hitched a red flannel nightingale to his skinny chest. There was a large hole in his throat.

The hole had been made by an anchor which was inconveniently dropped on the exact spot where Dummy had dived to collect a drunken bet. Fortunately the other sailors on his ship were still sober enough to miss him when he didn't come up and Dummy was hauled on deck in time for his life to be saved but too late to do much about his throat. It took him a long time to adjust to having no voice and a large hole where his throat should have been, and when he did he had nowhere to go and no one to go to, so he established himself for life in one of our side wards. He resisted all attempts to find a place for him somewhere else and after a while everybody stopped trying and he became a part of the building. And a very valuable part sometimes.

'Watch out for Dummy,' Baker said when I told her I was running on Male Two. 'He'll frighten you to death when you first see him, but he's lovely really.' He certainly was. He never seemed to need sleep. He stood at his window most of the night looking at us. If he noticed one of us dropping off when we should have been sitting upright and alert at the table he wandered into the ward and touched us on the arm, sending us rocketing to the ceiling with fright. If a patient became rude or difficult Dummy waited until he got a little too rude and a little too difficult, then he came in and with a few well-chosen grunts he put the offender in his place never to offend again.

It was Dummy who comforted me, and made innumerable cups of tea and lit innumerable cigarettes for me on the night, much later, when I found an empty bed where a patient should have been. He held up his flannel cape between me and the man swinging from the bathroom ceiling and kept it there until he had prepared me for what I had to look at. He grunted me into believing that I needn't feel guilty for the rest of my life for allowing one man to go his own way while forty-nine others were clamouring for my attention.

'Is he the same on days?' I asked Baker.

'He's worse,' she said. 'He goes round with the doctors and tells them what they ought to be doing.'

'How do they know what he's saying?' I asked.

'They don't, but the funny thing is if Dummy thinks a man could do with a bottle of Guinness with his supper he usually gets it.' I believed her. Dummy was able to get his message over loud and clear in spite of the disadvantage of having no vocal cords.

As well as sitting importantly at the table while our seniors sat drinking tea in the kitchen we had the added burden of relieving them for their main meal at midnight. They always went to the first sitting while the mince was still hot and plentiful. Before they went they gave us a list of dos and don'ts which, unless we carried them out properly, could get us into a lot of trouble when they came back. That first night mine was short and to the point.

'See that old Smith doesn't fall out of bed while I'm away. He's always doing it and he'll kill himself one of these nights. It had better not be tonight while I'm away. Don't bother to go to number five if he calls. He tries it on when the runner's left in charge. Just ignore him. If you get an admission, which God forbid, tell the porter to stick it in the middle bed till I get back. And for pity's sake, keep Freddy out of Dennis's bed.' Then off she went.

She seemed to think that keeping Freddy out of Dennis's bed was as important as old Smith killing himself by falling out of bed, though I had no idea why it could be that important.

Freddy had been in a long time and would never go out again though he was still barely thirty. The complaint he had took its time but got there in the end. Dennis had bright orange hair, a funny walk and a gentle way with him. He was in for some sort of hormone treatment. I asked him one night how he came to have orange hair. I was no wiser after he had finished telling me.

'Well, it's like this, you see. I live in Carlton and everybody there knows what I am.' He obviously thought I knew as well. I didn't.

'What are you?' I asked politely. He evaded the question after a quick look at me to see whether I was being serious.

'How did your hair get that colour?' I persisted.

'Well, it's like this, you see. Me mother got fed up with the neighbours talking so she chucked me out. Then I went up to London to be a female impersonator.'

'A what?'

'A female impersonator.'

'What's that?'

'Well, you know, one of them blokes what dresses up as a woman.'

'What on earth would he want to do that for?' I said, mesmerized. Again he evaded the question.

'I had to have me hair dyed blonde to be a female impersonator.'

'But it's not blonde, it's orange.'

'Yes well, I wasn't very good at being a female impersonator so they sacked me, then I started sinning for money. I didn't like sinning for money so I came back to Carlton and tried to dye me hair back again and this is how it went.' It all sounded very queer to me but I let it pass.

Dennis was a kind-hearted young man. While he was in, he was very good to Freddy. During the day, when sister was off, they went for walks together in the woods behind the ward. Baker told me that when they went the men used to give them a cheer and another when they came back. They always came back looking very happy, Baker said. Freddy was never the same again after Dennis went home, he missed the walks and the companionship, but at least he'd had them, which was more than he would have if Dennis had never come in.

That night he slept peacefully in his own bed and didn't need me to keep him away from Dennis, which was just as well. I had other things to think about.

The nurse in charge had only just disappeared down

the corridor when the porter brought up an admission. My heart sank. I was not prepared for such a weight of responsibility as an admission.

'Don't you worry about it,' said the porter kindly, 'I'll take him down and give him a good bath for you. He's a bit drunk but he'll sober up when he's had a bath. He's been in a fight by the looks of him.' The two of them walked down the ward to the bathroom. Within seconds the porter was back.

'I'm ever so sorry, Nurse, but I've come without a sponge bag. I'll have to go down to the porter's room for it. Nip up to the bathroom and keep an eye on the lad while I go.'

I stood in the bathroom and looked at the drunken boy with what I hoped was a pitiful expression of charitable tolerance. He looked back at me with the same wary suspicion. Neither of us said anything for a few minutes then at last he spoke.

'I suppose you think you're a bleeding angel then, do you?' He was quite right, except for one small detail. I didn't just think I was an angel, I knew I was. Either an angel of mercy, a ministering angel, or just any old plain celestial angel. I kept a dignified silence until the porter came back.

When we put him into bed the boy refused to lie down. He sat bolt upright watching me fussing importantly at the table. Then he called me over to him. He looked balefully round at the sleeping men and back to me.

'Are you by yourself here with all these blokes?' I nodded, not caring to explain that my trusteeship was only temporary.

'If any of them starts anything, you just wake me up and I'll look after you.' He gave the men another warning look then lay down and went to sleep.

Later in the night the police came and took him away with them. He seemed as surprised as I was when they told him he had murdered a man. I still think that without the drink he could have been a very nice boy. I also think that had any of the men started anything, which was highly unlikely, he would have looked after me.

If, in spite of my self-glorification, none of us were angels, we certainly bled. We bled constantly from wounds inflicted on us by whip-tongued sisters and staff-nurses, who bled from wounds inflicted upon them by the Matron and senior medical officers, who no doubt spent a lot of time licking their own wounds. But none of us bled too much for the patients. Early in our career sister-tutor had advised us against bleeding too freely for them. Before she started delving into the mysteries of anatomy and physiology she had given us her recipe for the makings of a good nurse.

'The function of a nurse is to care for the sick. A

good nurse will treat her patients with kindness and understanding, without ever getting too involved with their suffering. This detachment is often called hardness by those outside the profession. It is not hardness, it is our defence against being torn to emotional shreds by the work we are called upon to do. The nurse who bleeds for her patients will find herself bleeding in vain, she will get more reward from caring for them.'

Sister-tutor also had a few words to say on the makings of a good patient.

'It would be as hard to define a good patient as it is to define a good nurse. All of you at some time in your career will encounter mild old ladies who, in the sweetest way imaginable, can turn every nurse into a stubborn unyielding monster simply by asking for a handkerchief to be picked up. You will also encounter screaming viragos and ferociously cursing men who will have you eating out of their hands, and rushing willingly to anticipate their slightest wish. Good patients, like good nurses, are born, not made.' Our wise sister-tutor, she knew it all.

When the senior nurse strolled casually back from the mess-room after eating her mince, and had been told all about the new patient in the middle bed, I was allowed to tear across for my meal. Baker and Pickford were already there sharing their experiences with Davies.

'God,' said Pickford flopping across the table. 'That's been a bloody night that has.' We resisted the temptation to remind her that the night had still a long way to go before it could be talked about in the past tense. She started to giggle. We looked at her inquiringly.

'Well, there was this death on Male Chronic, you see. The sister made me go across to the morgue with it and Collington went with me. He's dafter than all the other porters put together. Halfway across one of the wheels fell off the trolley. Well naturally the body fell off as well. Collington and me tried to get it back on again. Then Collington's torch went out and he couldn't find the keys to the mortuary. So I had to stand and hold the trolley and the body while he went back to get another battery for his torch. It was awful. The body kept slipping and I kept having to shove it back on again, and the worst of it was it was huge.' She fell silent and we could see she was picturing the inky black grounds, no porter, and a body struggling to get off the three-wheeled trolley. We tried to picture it ourselves and fell over our mince laughing. Our attitude to death had already taken on a new dimension. We had begun to see it as a natural conclusion to living, unless the circumstances were too awful even for us to take a detached view.

Baker had been on Gynae. Her experience in the small theatre on the corridor quite put her off her mince and she only ate the rice pudding. We finished our meal and rushed back to our wards.

It was all waiting for me when I reported on duty. The nurse in charge ran through a string of things I had done wrong while she was away then I was permitted to go and get on with my work. 'And see you do it a bit better than you seem to do things when I'm away.'

'Yes, Nurse,' I said and scurried down to the sluice before she could think of any other way of reviling me.

Following the duty list minute by minute I cleaned and polished instruments, cleaned and polished sterilizers, filled drums, laid up trays and trolleys for the morning work, gave out bottles, gave out more bottles, collected specimens, boiled up specimens, helped my seniors with another round of tepid sponging, poulticing and making patients who were comfortable less comfortable. When the supply of work in the ward had been temporarily exhausted I went into the kitchen and started another lot.

I cut mounds of bread and marged the slices, clamping them together so firmly with damp tea towels to keep them moist that when breakfast-time came they would need to be prised apart with a knife, leaving one slice plastered with marge and the opposing slice with no marge on it at all. I clanked crockery, clattered cutlery, rattled teapots and dropped lids until even I was roused from my tiredness by the noise I was making.

I halved grapefruit for diabetics, after checking carefully that the diabetics were eligible for grapefruit, I put rashers of bacon in the hot plate to frizzle gently and eggs in saucepans of cold water ready to boil furiously. Then when it was all done I relieved my seniors for the full half hour it took each of them to eat their cob loaf and stood for a split second in one of the kitchens while I gobbled up what was left of mine.

And at four thirty the main lights in the ward were turned up, the little green cloths were unpinned and put away and the morning work began. From then until seven all was chaos. I rushed up and down the wards with bottles, bowls and bedpans and got annoyed when someone asked me for something different from what they were getting at that precise moment.

'Can I have a drink please, Nurse?'

'No you can't, it's bottle time now.'

'Can I have a bottle please, Nurse?'

'No you can't, it's washing time now.'

'Can I have a bowl please, Nurse?'

'I just gave you one.'

'Well you took it away again before I had time to have a wash.'

'Then you should have sat up and got washed before I took it away.'

'Can I have a clean towel please, Nurse?'

'You'll have to wait a minute.'

'But I've waited two days already.'

'Then another minute won't hurt you.'

When every patient either had or hadn't had a bottle, a wash-bowl, a bedpan and all the other things they craved for it was time to start giving out the breakfasts. Our cooking never reached cordon-bleu standard. The bacon we had put in to frizzle gently came out blackened or raw. The eggs we boiled collapsed at a touch or remained impervious to the stoutest hammering, and the toast we made as a special favour for the poorly ones was usually charred before they got it. The porridge that came up from the main kitchens already cooked had its own peculiarities. One of the duties of the runner between Female One and Female Two was to go over to the kitchens several times during the night and stir the porridge. The moment she turned the lights on hundreds of cockroaches sought sanctuary. Some fled behind waste pipes, some hid beneath sinks, others fell into the cauldrons of porridge, never to be seen again until a patient fished one out of his porridge bowl.

'Quick, Nurse, there's a cockroach in me porridge.'

'Well it's dead, isn't it?'

'Mebbe so, but I doan't fancy me porridge after there's been a cockroach in it.'

'You'll just have to do without your porridge then, won't you?' It was no use complaining to us, we had our own problems. We spent a lot of valuable time picking ants out of the tea caddy.

At seven o'clock the night was over, unless there had been a death at an inconvenient time that couldn't be put off for the day nurses, or an admission was brought in refusing to wait until we went off before he showed signs of collapsing, or we were kept behind by the day sister who had seen at a glance something we had left undone, or something we had done which we shouldn't.

'May I go off duty please, Sister?'

'Are the sluices tidy?'

'Yes, Sister.'

'Have you charted the specimens?'

'Yes, Sister.'

'Are all the breakfast things in?'

'Yes, Sister.'

'Then I suppose you can be dismissed.' And we dismissed ourselves fast before she found something we had to say 'No, Sister' to, and went across to the mess-room for yet another helping of mince and rice pudding.

Chapter Fourteen

OFFICIALLY WE GOT less free time on nights than we did on days. Apart from the night off a month – if we were lucky – all we had were 'evenings'. Once a week we were allowed to report on duty at eleven instead of nine. None of us cared much for these concessions. They did nothing to further our love-life, our social life, or any other life we might have wished to indulge in outside hospital hours. We usually spent our 'evenings' in bed, and having no Nelly to nag us awake, we overslept, arriving on duty hot and late and destined for the Matron's office in the morning.

It was after one of these doubtful privileges that I went on the ward and saw a set of screens arranged round a bed which could mean only one thing – a death.

The nurse in charge greeted me with the customary lack of warmth that the lower orders of probationer nurses quickly became accustomed to.

'You're never here when you're wanted, are you?' she

stormed. I agreed, hanging my head in shame at my remissness.

'Well now that you've at last condescended to come on duty you'd better go and lay up a trolley then come and help me behind the screens.'

I stared at her, aghast. I had never helped anyone in that way behind the screens before. On day duty such things were dealt with by nurses much senior to me.

'Get along then, and look sharp about it,' said the nurse. I got along.

When I had finished laying up the trolley and checked and re-checked its requirements I put on the gown and mask that were obligatory on these occasions. Then I pushed the trolley out and edged it and myself cautiously between the screens. The nurse was already busy with the preliminaries and didn't even look at me. Our seniors seldom did unless they were telling us off for something or other and even then they chose a spot somewhere in the middle distance to hurl their insults at. We worked quietly for a long time while I tried not to look at what we were doing or what we were doing it to. When the moment arrived for the final arraying the nurse glanced briefly over her mask.

'Shroud,' she barked in a controlled hiss. I jumped. The silence behind the screens had been so intense that her voice, hollow behind the mask, brought back all the fears that had kept me hovering outside the screens before I plucked up enough courage to get inside them. I stood transfixed. She again glanced briefly at me.

'Shroud,' she repeated. This time the hiss was a little less controlled. I looked at her and at the trolley and tossed everything about in a desperate attempt to locate the missing garment before the hiss developed into hysteria. When the nurse realized that there was nothing forthcoming in spite of her repeated request, she straightened up and glared at me. Her eyes above the mask grew round and angry.

'What's that you've got on?' she said, shaking with suppressed fury. I followed her gaze down my person and saw that in place of the severely tailored nurse's gown I should have been wearing I had on a ruched and ruffled creation that was clearly the missing shroud. I got out of it as fast as I could and gave it to her and we went on with our work.

When I told the others about it in the mess-room at midnight they refused to believe me at first.

'You're making it up,' said Weldon.

'God's honour,' I assured her.

'Was she livid?' asked Davies, convinced at last.

'Puce,' I replied. They mentally dressed me in a shroud and we laughed so much we were late back on the ward.

*

Night duty affected us all in different ways. It robbed Pickford of the curse she so desperately prayed for and had us praying for every month. Davies came out in a fresh crop of spots and so did I, just when we were starting to get rid of our last lot. As well as the spots I was afflicted by a terrible feeling of isolation. Sometimes when I was sitting at the table, it seemed to me as if I was the only one awake in the universe. Each tremendous heave across a bed made me long to be where the patients were, snug and warm between the sheets. That many of them were minus a leg or an arm or some other vital part of their anatomy did nothing to lessen my envy of them. Their mown-down pastures were infinitely more lush than my own unscythed grass. Each grunt and groan and gusty sigh only made things worse.

When these feelings got the better of me I looked for no spiritual help to lighten my darkness. I had already discovered a more earthly way out of my afflictions. All I needed to do whenever I had a minute to spare was to step out onto one of the verandahs.

The hospital stood at the junction of three roads. On the island in the middle of the junction there was a flashing orange light that had been put there by courtesy of Mr Hore-Belisha, whose name it took to posterity. There were many such beacons up and down the country. They had only just been thought up and were still something of a novelty, but none served a more useful purpose than that one did. It kept me sane when I was almost beside myself with itchy spots and loneliness. While the light continued to flash its friendly message, I could believe that someone besides me was alive and well, and would soon be ready to start the world moving again. I would dwell for as long as I had time for on an aunt of mine – the one that God had used to come between me and my mother's dislike of sewing – who declared that she never went to bed before three o'clock in the morning, and on my parents who were up again at five except on Sundays, then refreshed and fortified I went back to work again. The little trips to the verandahs had other uses as well as the therapeutic one.

Because of the even greater restriction of our off-duty on nights it was even more necessary to find ways and means of overcoming the problem. Any of us wishing to live a full and dangerous life while we were on night duty often found it easier not to go to bed at all, thereby allowing a whole day of glorious freedom. All that was needed was plenty of stamina and a gift for lying ourselves out of awkward situations when they arose. By the time we went on nights even the more dedicated ones had acquired a little of both.

When the mornings were golden and the dawn chorus was heady enough I went back into the ward and laid the foundations for one of these days of freedom. Davies was usually the first to be sounded, partly because she was still my closest friend and partly because she had a bicycle. The telephone call had to be made as slyly as the trips to the verandah were made. Either would have called the wrath of the nurse in charge down on my head if she had known about them.

'Hello, it's me, how about not going to bed today and going out instead?'

'How can we? Mary will catch us.'

'She won't if we're careful.'

'How will we get out?'

'We'll eat our mince first, then while Mary's busy with the post we'll nip up to our rooms and get changed, then sneak out the back and get our bikes out.'

'How will we get past the lodge-man?'

'We can dodge behind an ambulance or something and pedal through the big gates, instead of the side gate. He'll never see us.'

'You hope.'

'Oh for God's sake, if you don't want to come don't come …'

'It's not that, I just know I'll feel terrible tonight not having any sleep.'

'Oh don't bother, I'll ask Weldon.' Weldon was usually willing to take a chance on being caught either by Mary or the lodge-man, and she also had a bicycle. She was also not averse to going without sleep occasionally, however awful she might feel when she got on duty that night.

The reason I had a bicycle was because an exceedingly rich young man had sent me one after he had been attracted to my spots at one of the hospital balls. The spots were the only thing we had in common. He bustled about plying me with sausage rolls while I made nervous conversation. It was the first time I had talked to someone only three or four generations removed from a belted earl and the experience took a little while to get adjusted to. I tried very hard.

'What a beautiful evening,' I murmured, looking soulfully through the concert-room window. For all I knew it could have been raining cats and dogs.

'Quite enchanting,' he agreed. The talk lapsed while we ate several more sausage rolls and three-cornered sandwiches. Being both strictly teetotal we drank nothing but lemonade.

'Where do your people live?' he asked at last, wiping the crumbs off his starched front. I thought fast.

'They have a little place in the country,' I replied truthfully, making it sound as if 'little' was my modest way of describing a mansion. 'I miss it all so much since I left dear Papa and Mamma and came to be a nurse. I miss the song of the birds when I wake up in the morning, the rustle of spring and the wind on the heath.' I was thoroughly enjoying myself by this time. I went on. 'To be alone, all alone to commune with nature is all I ask.' Then I dried up.

'So like dear Miss Garbo,' he murmured.

'Pardon,' I said. I had never heard of the woman. The next day the bicycle arrived. It had my name on the handlebars, a letter stuck to the seat and a de luxe edition of *The Wind in the Willows* in the saddlebag with the repair outfit. The letter explained that the bicycle and the book were intended to foster my love for the great outdoors. And who knows, maybe they did.

Immediately after the bicycle arrived I got an urgent summons to the Matron's office. She gave me a frosty look when I went in.

'I believe you have just received a gift from the young man who was speaking to you at the ball last night?'

'Yes, Matron,' I said.

'I have sent for you to warn you against nurturing any romantic ideas about him. He is considerably above you in his station in life and it would be wise for you to forget him at once. You may keep the gift since he saw fit to send it to you, but I trust such a thing will not happen again.' I felt it was hardly likely to and as I left the office it occurred to me that until the bicycle arrived I hadn't given the giver a single thought. But in view of what the Matron had said about forgetting him I started thinking about him a lot, conjuring up visions of him carrying me off in his Silver Cloud and making me mistress of his broad acres.

The following Christmas we were invited to his country seat for tea, and went in relays. He didn't even recognize me for which I was grateful. The fuss they made over the hot cakes was bad enough without him rubbing salt in the wounds.

'Pass the hot cakes, dear,' his mother had said, looking disdainfully over my right shoulder. It took me a little while to realize she was talking to me and when I did I got very flustered. I behaved in much the same way as I had behaved while I was searching for the shroud, while liveried men and frilly-aproned serving girls watched me contemptuously. None of them came to my rescue and it was Pickford who eventually saved me from further disgrace. She also was above me in her station of life and knew about things like hot cakes. She lifted the lid off a huge silver dish and there they were, nestling together and keeping each other warm. We called them scones at home and ate them straight from the oven without the intermediary of a silver dish.

The incident ruined the outing for me and left the servants with a poor opinion of nurses.

Despite my assurances to Davies on the telephone, getting out early in the morning was as tricky as getting in late at night. Being broad daylight the railway embankment was no use to us and a different technique had to be employed. Weldon and I did it in exactly the way I had described it to Davies and soon we were pedalling furiously through the lodge gates.

Those days were memorable, being stolen. Sometimes we went to Newstead Abbey and trod in reverent silence the paths that had been trodden long ago by Byron and his unhappy lady loves. We sighed and sorrowed over the tomb of his faithful dog Boatswain, and we ate threepenny pork pies and drank fizzy lemonade while we tried to keep awake, and desperately tried to hide our yawns.

Sometimes we biked to Edwinstowe and stood marvelling at the Major Oak, which was tall enough and wide enough and hollow enough to shelter an army of runaway kings. Not to mention Robin Hood and all his merry men. And possibly Maid Marion as well, with the Sheriff of Nottingham thrown in for good measure.

Once I went on my own to Chesterfield, not to gaze at the crooked spire but to visit a promising romance who had sworn undying love while I was blanket bathing him one day. I should have learned my lesson the first time, when the passionate suitor behind the bathroom door lost all his passion as soon as he hit the fresh air, but I didn't. I sweated and pedalled my way to Chesterfield, confident of the rapturous welcome and the diamond engagement ring that would be waiting for me when I got there. There was neither. All there was was a lot of embarrassment on both sides. After a disappointing day when we could find nothing to say to each other something went wrong with my bicycle. I was due on duty at nine, it was already six and I had no money for train fares. I was desperate.

The boy, already yet another 'ex', whom I had gone twenty-six miles to see, felt he owed me something for my devotion and we rode all the way back to the hospital on his tandem. I had never ridden on a tandem before and the journey was punctuated with short halts while he replaced me with less and less tenderness on the back seat. We were well into Nottingham before it had sunk in that I was there to pedal the thing, not to steer it. I never saw him again. The ride back to Nottingham had proved conclusively, if he had needed any proof, that he was in no shape to carry me over a threshold. I even had to make my own arrangements for getting my bicycle back from Chesterfield.

Coming in through the gates in the evening was never too much of a problem. If the lodge-man saw us and questioned us we could always tell him we had got up and gone out after five when it was permitted but not encouraged. If Mary caught us we told her the same story. If neither of them believed us it was still their word against ours and they daren't make too much of it. Allowing us to get away in the morning without their catching us would have smacked of negligence if it had got as far as the Matron's office. After all what were they there for if they let us get away with things like that?

The thing that troubled us the most was the night that followed the day, when, as Davies was so ready to say 'I told you so', we felt awful with having no sleep. We started yawning the moment we got on duty and had to think up excuses for the yawns to satisfy our seniors.

'God, I'm tired. That bloody Nelly kept me awake all day with her scrubbing and her singing.'

'She didn't keep us awake,' pointed out the virtuous ones virtuously.

'It's all right for you, you sleep the other end of the corridor, she wasn't working there today.' They knew and we knew but we still battled it out.

While we were working, we went through different stages of tiredness, ranging from bursts of feverish activity bordering on hysteria, to a condition we called night nurse's paralysis. This was a trance-like stupor we all fell into at some time or another. It affected the good as well as the bad, though not perhaps as often. It happened in different places and took different forms. We could be sitting blamelessly at the table and see the night sister coming down the ward. Instead of leaping to our feet to pay her the homage that was her due we sat glued to the chair, our mouths opening and shutting like fish. She never sent us to the Matron when she found us in this condition; she waited until we had recovered then told us off herself.

A porter came across Weldon in the middle of the grounds one night. She had a bedpan in one hand and a sluice brush in the other and was singing 'A Policeman's Lot is Not a Happy One' at the top of her voice. It took the porter a long time to reason with her. She thought he was Harry, and being at the time of unsound mind she tried to take advantage of him. He told us afterwards that she was very insistent. She denied it all when we taxed her with it.

One night when I was sitting alone on Children's Medical, rolling swabs and packing drums, a gang of masked men burst in. Each one grabbed a baby and rushed off with it under his arm while I sat watching helplessly. I recovered from the paralysis and heard the babies still yelling for their bottles and not a masked man in sight. I had a momentary flash of disappointment. A gang of masked men would have been something to boast about in the mess-room.

Other pleasures we indulged in at the beginning of the month, while we still had money in our purses, were not as strenuous as the bicycle rides. We visited the more refined cafés in the town and occasionally went to a tea dance at the Palais. Sometimes we queued outside the Empire theatre – the Royal was beyond our means – and for sixpence, if we stood long enough and didn't mind standing again when we got in, we saw Gracie Fields or Bebe Daniels and Ben Lyon, and other celebrities of the day. Opposite the Empire there was a milk bar where we could sit and drink our raspberry milk shakes at the table next to them if we were lucky. We did a lot of name-dropping when this happened. It was as close as many of us would ever get to the famous.

The tea dances at the Palais were never very successful. There was too much competition. Nottingham was packed with beautiful girls, some earning as much as two pounds a week at Player's. They could afford to bleach their hair and buy lipstick. None of us could. And anyway the Matron would have frowned on both, especially the bleached hair. Even Pickford never went as far as that. There were other drawbacks to going to the Palais. We only went there to look for boy friends and if we happened to be lucky and get asked to dance we either had to rush off to be on duty, or else, not having much opportunity for dancing, we got our feet mixed up with our partners' and brought the foxtrot to a standstill. We were seldom invited for a second time round and we soon got discouraged and stopped going to the Palais altogether.

The visits to the cafés were much less competitive. In

the morning when we could afford it, if we were not too tired and if we hadn't got a lecture, we went to a coffee shop near the bus station and drank Russian tea from tall glasses with bits of lemon hanging down the side. None of us liked it much, and it was a long time before we knew what to do with the lemon, but it looked well and we were always anxious to be seen doing the things that looked well. It was also very lady-like, which would have made my mother happy.

At one of the cafés we went to there was a very poor three-piece string ensemble. I fell heavily in love with the violinist. He was thin and romantic-looking, and every time he tucked his violin under his chin I shivered. He remained unaware of my burning passion for a long time, then at the cost of several cups of tea I made him aware of it by throwing tender glances at him and giving him inviting little smiles. Cornered as he was between the potted plants and the piano there was no escape for him and one afternoon he came across and sat down at my table. This was a great pity. For a long time I had been happy suffering the tortures of unrequited love, but the moment he came out from behind the palms I began seeing the flaws. Without his violin and at close quarters he was an insignificant little man in a shabby, threadbare, swallow-tail coat, and boots that had seen better days. My heart sank. It sank even further when he accepted my offer of a cup of tea and drank it while he showed me snaps of his wife and kiddies taken in various poses outside their back door. After that I only went to the café when I could be sure he wasn't there. But I sadly missed the romantic violinist I had fallen so heavily in love with.

Baker was a vegetarian when she wasn't too hungry to be one. She insisted on taking us to a health-food store and restaurant, where we were given a nut cutlet and a very small helping of chocolate blancmange with a dab of vegetarian cream on it. While we ate it she tried to talk us into becoming vegetarians, but the nut cutlet put us off. The Irish girl tried to talk us into being Roman Catholics, but there were things about that which put us off. In the end we all gave up trying to persuade the others to be what we were, and were a lot happier for it.

Our regular eating habits were solved by a small dirty café in a small dirty back street where, on our days and nights off when we were not going home, we were able to get a substantial meal at a price we could afford. The food was homely if nothing like any of us had ever got at home. There was egg and chips, bacon and chips, sausage and chips, and different permutations of all three. In the event of us being too poor to afford any of these luxuries we were never sent empty away. The proprietor was fond of nurses he said, and couldn't do enough for them, and besides, as he pointed out, you never knew when you might be ill yourself and in the infirmary so it was just as well to keep in with the nurses. He laughed convulsively at his joke and we laughed with him.

He was big and fat, and wore a set of greasy overalls that might once have been white, but that was a long time ago. He did everything himself including the washing up, and we tried not to notice the smudges of second-hand mustard round the edge of the plates. If we were completely destitute he would make us a sausage sandwich and allow us to owe him for it until we were not so broke. His sausage sandwiches were mouth-watering masterpieces. He made each one before our very eyes. He threw a couple of sausages into a pan, already well greased and blackened from the previous lot of sausages, gave them a quick sizzle on all sides, slapped them on a slice of bread, threw half a bottle of sauce over them, slapped another slice of bread on top, gave it all another friendly slap and handed it over the counter to us in his fingers.

When it was Mannering's birthday we decided to celebrate the occasion by going to the small dirty café. Mannering was a class below us but we liked her a lot. She had earned our respect by the speed she learned to slide down the railway embankment. She was always game for an illicit day out and knew more ways of avoiding Mary and foxing the gate-porters than many a nurse years her senior.

None of us had much money to celebrate with but when we explained to the proprietor that it was Mannering's birthday he made a special effort to make the day a memorable one. In this he succeeded beyond our wildest dreams. He put three sausages in her sandwich instead of the customary two and gave it a couple of extra slaps for luck. When it was finished he had to undo it all again because he had forgotten the sauce. Finally he held it up for our inspection and declared modestly that it was the finest sausage sandwich he had ever made. He watched Mannering eat it with a smile of justifiable pride on his face.

At midnight she came to the mess-room looking very peculiar.

'What's the matter with you?' we asked her.

'It's my stomach,' she groaned, pushing aside the mince.

'What's wrong with your stomach?'

'It bloody well hurts.'

'Have you told the night sister?'

'Yes, but she said I couldn't go off sick. I'm on Gynae and we're busy.' Mannering groaned again and went back to Gynae.

Like my mother, the night sister didn't believe in illness, especially when it affected her staff and made her short of nurses. She waited until Mannering collapsed at her feet before she sent her across to her room.

'I hope you're not malingering, Nurse.'

'No, Sister, I'm not.'

'Well then, I suppose you'd better go to your room. I'll send somebody across to have a look at you later.' Unfortunately she forgot and by the time we went off duty poor Mannering was past being looked at.

When we came out of quarantine the small dirty café had been shut down. We missed it and the fat jolly proprietor that went with it. We never did pay him what we owed him for the celebration sausage sandwiches.

Chapter Fifteen

WHEN WE WERE told we were to be in charge of wards of our own the shock almost made patients of us. Though it was our second time round on nights the thought of being responsible for the lives of more than forty patients with nobody to lean on if we got into difficulties filled us with dread. Baker was the first to know. She came tearing across the mess-room to tell us.

'My God, guess what, I'm going on Female San on my own.'

'You're not.'

'I bloody am.'

'My God.' When it came to my turn the night sister seemed to have serious doubts, then sighing deeply she took the plunge.

'Male Three,' she said. 'In charge.' I blanched.

'What, me?' I said, caught off balance for a moment.

'Yes, you,' she said. 'You've passed your prelim haven't you?'

'Yes, Sister,' I said aloud. 'But only just,' I added under my breath, and it had been hard work.

Somewhere between running up and down the ward at the beck and call of our seniors and the patients, doing our bit of courting in the back seat at the pictures instead of watching *The Shape of Things to Come*, sipping our Russian tea and eating our nut cutlets, we somehow found time to study for our exams. Some of us more diligently than others as the exam results would clearly show. As at school, we learned many things we would never need to know and were left in ignorance of things that might have been useful to us. We painstakingly traced the passage of sewage from the lavatory pan back to the kitchen sink, paying a call to a sewage farm in order to get the proper feel of the thing. We earnestly studied the conversion of mare's milk into human mother's milk, though for what purpose was never made clear to us. We learned how to put leeches on and how to drop salt on their tails to get them off again. All the leeches we ever saw were safely screwed down in test tubes and had been for a long time. They were as obsolete as cupping, blood-letting and turpentine stupes, but we spent hours learning how to deal with them.

We put things into patients and took things out of them. We poulticed, purged, plastered and posseted. We gave hot baths, cold baths, starch baths and bran baths.

We made air beds, water beds, comfortable beds and not-so-comfortable beds. We studied organs, bones, sinews and blood vessels, where they had come from, where they were going and what they had been put there for in the first place. We practised lifting people up and laying them down – and out – without doing them or ourselves a mortal injury. It was all a question of knack, said sister-tutor, and never brute force. For a long time the brute force came easier than the knack, though the knack would have saved us many an aching back, and our patients much discomfort. They suffered while we learned.

And at the end of eighteen months we sat for our prelim, and either failed or passed according to the time we had spent with our books, or with Ernest and Bertha in the lecture room.

Ernest had been dead for a long time, and looked it. He dangled from a wardrobe, his dry bones doing a *danse macabre* whenever a door was opened. Bertha was blonde and buxom and made of rubber. She was so lifelike that a window cleaner took pity on her one day and complained to the authorities about the patient in the side ward who was not getting the treatment she deserved. He had to be allowed in to pinch her himself before he was convinced that she wasn't real. We did things to Bertha long before we were efficient at doing them to live ladies and she bore it all with fortitude.

I collected my night nurse's basket and reported to Male Three. The sister was no happier at seeing me than I was at being there.

'Have you passed your prelim?'

'Yes, Sister.'

'Have you been in charge of a ward before?'

'No, Sister.'

'Why are you in charge tonight then?' A good question. 'Please, Sister, I think it is because night sister is short of seniors.'

'Have you given injections?'

'Yes, Sister.' I thought it best not to tell her that I had only given injections to Bertha and even her rubber bottom didn't look the same afterwards.

'Well, I suppose you'll have to do,' she said doubtfully. 'I'll take you round the ward.' She did, and at every bed we came to I grew more frightened. I could feel my inexperience breaking through and showing itself to the men. We stopped beside one of the cot-beds. The man in it smiled at the sister and scowled at me. 'This is a new nurse, dad,' she bellowed at him. 'She will be giving you your injection tonight.' The man looked at me with hatred.

'I want no bloody new nurse doing her practising on me. Tell her to go and practise on someone else. I've had enough o' them wenches sticking needles in me backside and not knowing half the time where they're sticking 'em.' I thought of poor Bertha's mutilated bottom and knew how he must be feeling.

We passed down the ward.

The sister's face grew softer as we leaned over the next bed. The patient's face was engraved with blue pit lines.

'Hello, Bill, we've got a new nurse for you tonight. If you ask her nicely she might scratch your legs for you when they start itching.' Bill looked at her gratefully as we walked away, while she told me about him.

'Bill hasn't got any legs, Nurse. He lost them in a pit disaster but he doesn't believe it. They get itchy in the night when his injection wears off, then he can't get to sleep again until someone goes and scratches them for him. It's no good telling him he hasn't got any legs. He won't believe you, so you might just as well save your breath and humour him a bit.' I made a mental note of Bill's itchy legs so that I wouldn't forget to humour him when the need arose.

There were two screens round one of the beds and as I followed the sister through them a huge red-headed man sat crouched as if ready to spring on us. The sister touched him gently on the shoulder and he relaxed on the pillows.

'All right, Mac, it's only me. I'm bringing the new nurse round, she's not going to bite you.' I felt there was more chance of him biting me, then I saw that he was blind: he also had a tube in his throat that was held firmly in place by a bandage. He put his fingers to the tube and spoke to me. His voice was thick and guttural with a heavy Scots accent.

'Good evening, Nurse,' he said politely. 'Ye'll no' forget ma Guinness, will ye?' I promised and we went on our way.

'You'll have to keep an eye on him, Nurse. He's been a bit depressed today and when he's depressed he tries to take the trachy tube out and kill himself.'

'Why has he got one in?' I asked.

'He got drunk after a football match and someone cut his throat with a bottle. He lost his sight after a football match as well, he always gets drunk when his team loses. He gets drunk when they win but not as bad as when they lose. He's lucky to be alive.' And so was I one night. Mac was a lovely man until his depression got the better of him, then he struggled and fought to tear the tube out of his throat, which would have meant instant death. He almost managed it once when there was only me on the ward to keep his hands off it. After he had calmed down and stopped trying to strangle me he offered me one of his boiled sweets and apologized for his anti-social behaviour. I accepted both the sweet and the apology.

We finished the round and after a lot of final instructions the sister went off duty, giving the ward a last lingering look as though she never expected to see it looking like that again.

I spent the next few minutes injecting water into a pillow to brush up my technique and when the time came for me to try out my skills on human flesh instead of on rubber and feathers I approached the old man somewhat timidly. He glared at me all the way down the ward.

'Get away from me,' he roared. 'I want none of your bloody pins in me.' I wasn't too happy about it either, but I pulled his sheet down and his nightshirt up and got on with the job. When I had finished he chuckled happily. 'Fine bloody new nurse you are,' he chortled. 'You've done that a few times I know.' I hadn't, but it was nice to think he thought so. It gave me more confidence for the next time.

As well as practising my new-found skills on the patients I practised my new-found rank-pulling on the runner. I made her life a misery. I bellowed at her and bawled at her and bullied her, directed her and misdirected her, made her fetch and carry for me and treated her so shockingly that the poor girl didn't know where she was. I was crazed with power. It was lovely. I got back on her for all the things I had been made to suffer while I was a runner, just as eventually she would get back on someone for the tortures I put her through. Little did she know that it was all one big bluff.

However junior we still were when we were put in charge of a ward, we were expected to be able to cope. Whatever situation arose, whether we had met it before or not, whether sister-tutor had expounded on it in the lecture room or not, we were expected to deal with it calmly and competently, showing none of the panic we might be feeling. Often we had only the vaguest idea of what we should be doing but we did it, using the little knowledge we had and as much common sense as we were blessed with, and if we were lucky, which by the grace of God we usually were, the patient came through the ordeal still breathing, or at least persuaded by us that the agony he thought he was suffering wasn't really agony at all but a little thing that would go away when he had drunk a nice cup of warm Ovaltine. We relied a lot on Ovaltine in those days. It was cheaper than drugs and a lot less habit forming.

The night would have been a quiet one if it hadn't been for Bill's legs and the boy who was brought in at midnight nearly bleeding to death.

Bill's legs were a terrible trial to him. During the day he was a model patient, the wit of the ward (every ward has one) and a joy to nurse. But at night he was a different man. The moment the lights were dimmed the legs he had left behind in a pit one day screamed in agony at the indignities they had been made to suffer.

'For Christ's sake, somebody, will you come and

scratch me legs,' shouted Bill. And whoever was the nearest would spend a moment or two scratching the empty spaces where the legs should have been. For a while there would be peace then Bill started again. 'Will somebody come and cut me legs off before they drive me mad.' He was a lot happier when Tommy was brought in. Tommy was seventeen. He was brought in by half a dozen of his mates who knew he was dying and had clubbed together to give him a night out in Nottingham, determined that he should live a little before he died. Ungratefully he almost ruined the evening for them by bursting a blood vessel somewhere between Trent Bridge and Carlton. He had his blood transfusion and we put him into the empty bed next to Bill. For the next few weeks he hopped in and out of bed doing Bill's scratching for him and when he was too weak to hop in and out he and Bill comforted each other. The boy was as witty as Bill and as brave.

'Still alive then, sirrah?' he would say the moment he opened his eyes in the morning.

'Only just,' groaned Bill.

'What are you having for your breakfast?'

'Porridge with bloody cockroaches floating in it.'

'Never mind, mate, we'll both be as dead as them soon.' And they were.

It was when night sister moved me on to Male Two that one of the men got fed up with trying to guess what was wrong with him, and fed up with the doctor's evasive answers to his questions, and suspended himself from the bathroom ceiling with his dressing-gown cord. There had to be a post-mortem to make up the doctor's mind for him and I was got up in the middle of the afternoon one day to attend it. It was an experience that I could have well done without.

The dissecting was done in a small stuffy room that had no windows in it. The doctor who did it was tall and languid with a Ronald Colman moustache and a monocle that swung on a slim gold chain whenever he bent over a patient. He also had a limp which none of us believed was genuine. We thought he put it on with the monocle to impress everybody. He had a biting tongue which he used on the nurses more than anyone else. He had no illusions about their angelic vocation and saw them for what he considered them to be, scheming conniving females. Most of the time he was right. Once, when he was examining a temperature chart on one of the chronic wards, he screwed his monocle in his eye and scanned the undeviating tram lines under the headings of temperature, pulse and respiration, then he turned to his audience and drawled his opinion of them.

'Whenever one looks at a chart on a chronic ward, there springs to mind an irresistible picture of the night nurse sitting with her feet up on the table, a cigarette in her mouth and a cup of tea at her elbow taking the temperatures, while her patients lie undisturbed in their beds.' As a matter of fact we never sat with our feet on the table – we had all been brought up too nicely for that – we stuck them up on another chair while we went round every chronic with our mind's eye, assessing the heat of their blood, the rate of their heart beats and the depth of their breathing. These varied so little over the years that it was perfectly safe to put them down from memory except where pneumonia had set in, knocking everything haywire. By using our amazing powers of observation we were able to fore-cast the likelihood of this happening while we were doing the routine bottom-scouring. We were too familiar with the signs and symptoms of pneumonia to miss one of them.

As well as being cursed with a caustic wit Dr Dean felt the cold a lot. Before he started on a post-mortem he insisted on having a huge crackling fire burning in the small stuffy room. As an added insurance against the cold he did his work muffled to the ears in a top coat and a college scarf. Just in case this wasn't enough to keep the chill out of his bones he carried a silver flask in his hip pocket which he attacked at intervals while he was sorting out the bits he wanted to look at. He also liked to have a gramophone going at full blast somewhere in the room, presumably to keep his mind from dwelling too much on the task at hand. It was part of my duties to keep the gramophone wound up and see that there was plenty of coal on the fire. Dr Dean also fancied himself as a raconteur. When he wasn't taking swigs from the flask or humming out of tune with the gramophone he told us little stories of other gruesome ends he had been called upon to unravel in his time. As the flask got emptier the stories got nastier until one by one his audience started falling away. The live audience anyway, and the other was already past caring. I stayed on longer than I might have done if I hadn't been used to seeing buckets of offal lying about our kitchen at pig-killing time.

Another thing that imprinted the doctor on our memory long after he went was his passionate belief in the efficaciousness of garlic to cure all chest complaints. If a patient was coughing on the Sanatorium wards he got massive doses of cough mixture laden with garlic. If he wasn't coughing he still got it. Garlic was nature's own miracle worker according to Dr Dean, no matter what particular miracles happened to be needed. Garlic also discouraged the visitors on the wards that Dr Dean visited.

The children got it as well.

'Say ninety-nine like a very good child,' he would murmur to them softly.

'Ninety-nine like a very good child,' they would

answer, mesmerized by the swinging monocle, and he would pat them on the shoulder and go away satisfied that, with a few drops of disguised garlic night and morning, whatever they came in with would be gone by the time they went out. And sometimes it had.

Chapter Sixteen

FROM THE FIRST time we went on nights as trembling runners to the time we came off swollen-headed at being in charge of our own wards there had been a lot of changes around the place. Some good, some not so good.

Much to our own relief and sister-tutor's astonishment we had all passed our prelim. Ours had never been a particularly brilliant class. There were too many diversions, what with Pickford and the male nurses, but we had managed to scrape through and were well on the way to sitting for our finals.

We had reached the top of the second table in the mess-room and were getting some of our bread cut for us by the menials beneath us – God help them.

Nothing seemed quite as threatening and nothing quite so dire. There were still plenty of fleas on our backs to bite us but we bled less from their bites. Having done a bit of shrieking and shouting ourselves we had become less vulnerable to the shrieks and shouts of our seniors. We were uppish at being asked for a bedpan and well versed in the art of sending a raw recruit off in a rush to get it. With one imperious wave of the hand we were able to reduce a new probationer almost to tears just as we had been almost reduced to tears when we were new probationers. We were given no quarter then and we gave none now.

We listened with only half an ear to the Matron's scathing comments on our laziness, inefficiency and general unsuitability to be nurses. We had heard it all before and would again, and knew that we would go out of the office in one piece with no bloody teeth marks to show for the interview.

We came in late more often and got better at it, or we mended our ways through boredom or lack of the necessary stimulus and came in at the proper time via the bedding plants and the front door, taking in the gate-porter on the way. By this time I was able to reel my name off without any hesitation.

We had learned to placate Nelly and keep the ward maids' tale-telling mouths shut with a few cigarettes or a cheap bottle of scent at Christmas. We knew enough about their less desirable habits to be able to bribe and corrupt them until it was more than they dare do to go to the sisters about us. It was the survival of the fittest and we had become very fit over the past two years.

In the lecture room we were studying surgery and

medicine instead of anatomy and physiology, and the science of drugs instead of the meanderings of sewers and drains. I had been happier with sewers and drains: they carry less responsibility for a nurse. That is if you discount things like typhoid fever. Never having been much good at arithmetic the pressures involved in weighing, converting and administering dangerous drugs gave me more headaches than all the sewage farms in Nottinghamshire. Being asked to reduce the strength of a quarter of a grain of morphia, or something even more lethal, to an eighth by dissolving a tablet of the stuff over a bunsen flame then adding a drop or two of water until the desired dosage was reached was so primitive for everybody and so impossible for me that it was a miracle we weren't killing people all the time. The difference between the sign for a teaspoonful, and the sign for a tablespoonful was such a small squiggle it was the easiest thing in the world for it to get lost among all the other small squiggles the doctors littered the case sheets with. The patient who flinched at the thought of a fish-hooked needle penetrating his tender flesh would have done better to flinch at the thought of a nervous nurse getting her fractions wrong, or her squiggles mixed up. Those who did, and hit the headlines, paid dearly for an error which under other circumstances might have caused no more inconvenience than an unbalanced balance sheet. There is a far greater margin for error when people are dealing with numbers rather than lives.

If our education had progressed our ranks had been reduced. Strickland had drunk her Lysol in pitiful protest at being robbed of a friend, and Mannering, who loved life, had lost it because of the friendly gesture from the fat café owner. Pickford, too, had gone, but not so irrevocably, and was no doubt driving some other poor man to thoughts of murder or suicide with her beauty and her fickleness. And for the rest of us there had been changes, if not as traumatic, just as important to us.

Weldon was busily embroidering guest towels when she should have been studying, and listening to the distant patter of tiny feet when she should have been taking temperatures. Harry was spending less and less time in the parlour and more and more in the shed at the bottom of the garden knocking up coffee tables and three-piece suites. Poor Eric had gone the way of Strickland and Mannering. He had taken fright when his latest jilted girl friend threatened him with breach of promise unless he married her before the baby was born: he escaped to Spain and never came back, and the baby was born with a dead hero for a father instead of no father at all, which would make things a lot easier for it when it grew up.

The Irish girl had at last come into her fortune, though it was a long time before it did her any good. The news came when we were in the library one morning, smoking like chimneys and paving the way for lung cancers and coronaries before we were ninety. We heard her shrieking and rushed across to find out what was wrong with her.

'Holy Mother of God,' she yelled, waving a piece of paper about, 'I've come into a bloody fortune.' We stared at her disbelievingly. 'I've won the bloody sweepstake,' she said, looking round wildly for somewhere to collapse on.

When we had all had a good look at the piece of paper and counted the noughts we sat the Irish girl down on the floor and lit a cigarette for her. She had already got one in her mouth but we were too far gone by that time to notice. It was a long time before she recovered enough to say anything more, then, when she had stubbed out both cigarettes on the lino, she looked round us all.

'We'll dodge Mary and go to the Kardomah and celebrate,' she said generously.

'What will we celebrate with?' we asked the heiress. It was three weeks past the last pay day and a week before the next was due; none of us had a penny to bless ourselves with. We racked our brains, we plunged down chairs, we thought of pawn shops, and all to no avail and eventually we gave up the idea and went to bed. By the time pay day came round it was too late anyway. The Irish girl had lost her zest for celebrating and never really got it back. The thought of all that money lying in wait for her put her off her food and kept her awake at night for a long time. Like Lydia when she sat down on the cracked chamber-pot she was never the same girl again.

It was soon after that that Davies and I had our dreams of riches. None of them came to anything – financially at any rate. Davies did better than I did but in a way she never expected.

Being a municipal hospital there was no private block for paying patients. If the rich wanted to be ill they had to be ill in a nursing home or in one of the voluntary hospitals. If they were not really rich but looked as if they had been sometime, or there were other reasons why they preferred to come to us, then they were put into a side ward and were specialled by one of us. They got as good as they would have got in a nursing home but perhaps a little more boiled cod and plum duff. We nursed them just as conscientiously and they recovered or died at the same rate, without having to pay through the nose for the privilege. When a millionaire came into us because he was a socialist at heart despite his millions, and a City Father to boot, I was given the job of specialling him. I did everything for him, down to the most intimate. I bathed him and fed him, applied methylated spirits to his wrinkled old bottom and made cotton wool cushions for his wrinkled old other parts. I petted him, pampered him, and tried not to think of how rich he was. The others thought about it all the time. They drafted and redrafted his will a dozen times.

'He'll leave you thousands when he dies,' prophesied Davies hopefully.

'But he's not going to die,' I gloomed.

'He might,' said Weldon, encouragingly. 'After all he's not far off ninety.'

'And as strong as a horse,' I reminded her. They thought about it for some time, then Baker had a vision. She often had visions but most of them were too far-fetched to carry any credence.

'I can see it all,' she said, looking into the distance and seeing it all. 'It'll be all right, you'll see. The day he goes home he'll look at you with tears in his eyes and go down on his bended knees and thank you for saving his life.' When Baker wasn't courting Dr Collins she sat around reading things like *Peg's Paper*, where people were always going down on their bended knees.

'Once he's down on his knees he'll never get up again,' I said, 'and besides, I won't have saved his life, he only came in with gout.' They dismissed my protest as a bit of false modesty and Davies carried on where Baker left off.

'When he eventually gets off his knees he'll take out his cheque book—'

'And borrow your fountain pen,' broke in Weldon, 'and write you a cheque big enough to keep you in comfort for the rest of your life.'

'And us as well,' said Baker, thinking of Dr Collins, who would never make Harley Street. The Irish girl kept quiet. She still wasn't eating and knew only too well the miseries that riches brought in their wake.

Things didn't go quite the way they had planned them for me. On the day the old man went home his gentleman's gentleman and his liveried chauffeur came to collect him. They swathed him in furs and glossy astrakhan and tenderly led him to the waiting limousine, while I brought up the rear with an armful of bedpans and things the hospital had lent him to save him squandering his millions on them. The chauffeur flung open the door and the gentleman's gentleman loaded the precious cargo into the car, then he snatched the hired equipment off me and away they purred to their castle. The old man never looked my way. I walked sadly back to the ward with no bended knees and no cheque either.

'Mean old devil,' said Davies when I told her. 'Serve him right if he drops a bedpan on his other foot and gets gout in that as well.' I felt very bitter about man's ingratitude to nurses until I remembered the book and the bicycle, then I cheered up. If such a comparatively small offering could cause the Matron so much unhappiness and me so much trouble I shuddered to think how she would have reacted to my coming into thousands. She had been very cold about the Irish girl's windfall, she would have liked her to give it all back to the sweepstake people, but the Irish girl drew the line at that.

The patient that Davies specialled was no crusty old man but a charming old lady with a nose like a Roman emperor, and two daughters who sat in the side ward most of the time wearing silk-fringed shawls and smoking scented cigarettes from jewelled holders. They were clearly of the aristocracy. Davies had to put on a clean cap and apron and polish her shoes every morning. She told us that the daughters were lovely but they were driving her mad. They panicked every time she turned her back. She only had to go to the lavatory for one of them to come hammering at the door, which gave her terrible constipation she said.

'Darling Nurse,' they shouted frantically, 'do please hurry, darling Mother has taken a turn for the worse.' Or they would gaze at the still figure in the bed and implore Davies to tell them if darling Mother still lived. Davies said she got fed up assuring them that she did, though it was hard to tell sometimes.

For the first few weeks we spent Davies's thousands just as she had spent mine. Then suddenly she got huffy and told us all to shut up. She had grown attached to the old lady and her daughters and refused to consider anything as ignoble as taking money off them. She was adamant about it.

'Not a penny piece,' she maintained.

'But they'll insist,' we assured her, 'after all your constipated nursing.'

'It wouldn't matter, I still wouldn't take it.' And we believed her though she never got a chance to prove it. On the day the daughters shrieked, 'Darling Mother has gone,' and she had, Davies came off duty and cried. When she had finished crying she started to laugh. At first she refused to tell us why she was laughing, there seemed something not quite right in joking about things while the old lady was still under our roof as it were, but when she eventually told us we laughed as well. Nobody could have helped laughing.

'I did it all beautifully,' Davies told us. 'The old lady looked better after I had finished with her than she did before. Then when I'd done it all I went and asked her daughters if they wished to go and pay their last respects to her.' That was how we had been taught to do things by sister-tutor.

'When they came out,' went on Davies, 'I could see at a glance that something wasn't right for them. It wasn't just their mother being dead, it was something else but I didn't know what. So I asked them. "Is there something wrong?" I said. They held on to each other and looked at me in a sorrowful sort of way then the older one told me what it was. "Darling Nurse," she said, "when we were in the cubicle with our dear mother we couldn't help but notice that her bloomers were still on the chair. We feel you should know that she was the daughter of an archbishop and it would not be right for her to go to her grave with no bloomers on."' Davies paused for breath.

'What did you do?' we asked.

'What do you think I did?' she said. 'It took me ages.'

'What were they like?' we asked, wiping the tears from our eyes.

'Pink artificial silk with elastic everywhere.' We wore wide-legged French ones when we could afford them. They would have been a lot easier to get on. 'It was worth it though,' she said. 'You should have seen the look of gratitude on their faces when they went back to have a peep.'

When it had been written about in *The Times*, and the guest list gone over, the girls asked Davies for tea one day. When she came back she was full of it.

'They aren't a bit rich. I bet they haven't got a bean. They live in this marvellous cottage simply covered with some sort of ivy. The cottage I mean, not them.

They go about in dressing gowns with dragons down the back and there's something they call a samovar that they keep bubbling on the hob. The tea out of it tasted awful.' What she didn't tell us was that there was also a nephew. She didn't tell us about him for a long time and when she did she started getting very boring about him. Soon she was embroidering towels and comparing engagement rings with Weldon and Baker. I began to feel very left out, which was why I made such a dreadful mistake at the next Christmas ball.

The Christmas balls were very grand affairs. Everybody who was anybody turned up, the women in silks and satins and the men trailing behind them looking like sheepish nuns. None of us wore silks and satins. We wore cheap taffeta frocks that swept the floor unevenly on all sides or barely reached our ankles. Because the Christmas ball was held too soon after Christmas for our financial situation to recover we had no money for silk stockings or silver evening shoes so we went in our black woollen heavy-duty ones and our ward shoes, and spent the evening tugging and pulling at the straining taffeta trying to get it far enough down to cover our feet.

Before the ball started we rushed in and out of each other's rooms to have things done to our hair that seldom improved it, and to be assured that we did indeed look lovely.

'Does this dress look all right?'

'Of course it does. You just need a pin in the hem to keep it up.'

'Can you see the hole in my stocking heel?'

'Only when you walk.'

'I feel awful.'

'You look ever so nice.' We didn't believe it but it gave us fresh heart.

The band in the concert room played dreamy waltzes, languorous tangos and lively Charlestons, none of which we knew the first thing about. Our sessions at the Palais had done nothing at all for our sense of balance or rhythm. Apart from which only Davies had a partner. Evening dress was obligatory rather than optional and both Harry and Dr Collins were saving too hard to want to waste money on hiring them, so they stayed away. All of us except Davies sat round the walls trying to keep from under the dancers' feet. We took it in turn to weave in and out to the buffet tables at the opposite end of the room from the band.

The food was marvellous. It always seemed that the hospital cooks got so frustrated all the year turning out the horrible things that were expected of them that when it came to Christmas they let themselves go. They made tiny vol-au-vents that really did go with the wind, delicious savouries, creamy cakes, sherry-laden trifles and so many other fantastic concoctions that it seemed a pity to eat them, but eat them we did, almost without stopping. When our piled-up plates were empty we went and piled them up again. While it was there it had to be made the most of; there would be nothing like it for another year.

We carefully avoided the punch. The visitors were welcome to it. It was the Matron's speciality; only she knew its ingredients but we had examined it closely at one of the less important hospital functions.

'Cascara,' said Davies, sniffing at the brown sludge in a glass bowl.

'And cough mixture,' contributed Baker.

'With a few aniseed balls thrown in,' hazarded Weldon.

'And not a drop of whiskey,' lamented the Irish girl.

It was while I was downing my second plateful that I took my eyes off the food for a moment and saw a young man bearing down on me. I hastily removed a half-eaten sausage roll from my mouth, put the lemonade glass under the chair with all the other empties and sat and waited. I could feel the rings of sweat under my arms getting bigger.

'May I have the pleasure of this dance?' said the young man, bowing politely. I was flabbergasted. To be asked to dance was the last thing any of us expected at the dances. We were never prepared for the ordeal.

'I'm sorry but I'm afraid I can't do this one,' I said.

Evelyn Prentis

I had no idea which one it was but whichever it was I knew I couldn't do it. The young man refused to take no for an answer.

'It's only a foxtrot,' he said. 'All you have to do is follow me.' It was worse than riding the tandem. After I had steered him firmly round the room twice, there was a loud ripping noise.

'I'm terribly sorry,' I said, 'but I think you are standing on my dress.' He got off it and we edged our way back to the chair while he shielded my exposed rear end with his hands. Then we sat while he told me all about himself.

His name was Reginald, but that was only a quarter of it, the other three were equally distinguished. His mother was a widow and the Matron of a large hospital somewhere in the North. He was her only child. This was to become very apparent during the months that followed.

The reason he was at the ball was because he was something important down at the workhouse and had ambitions to be something even more important as soon as possible. He could also afford evening dress.

By the time the band played 'God Save the King' it had begun to dawn on me that he was mine if I wanted him. I didn't particularly want him but I knew only too well that time was running out for me. I was already turned twenty and had never embroidered a guest towel in my life, besides which an engagement ring would give me something in common with Weldon, Davies and Baker who were fast growing away from me. When he had finished standing strictly to attention for the national anthem he gave me my chance.

'If you are off on Sunday afternoon perhaps you would care to come to the Castle Art Gallery and look at the pictures, then we could have a crumpet in Lyons and afterwards go to church.' I took the chance without much enthusiasm.

Life with Reginald was duller than life with Harry had been, with no Eric to leaven the bread. We met at the same time in the same place every other Sunday and proceeded in an orderly fashion to the Castle Art Gallery. Neither of us knew anything about art but we spent many hours proving to each other that we did. There was only one picture in the whole collection that I thought anything of. It was a huge canvas that took up all one wall. On it there was a man in what appeared to be his shirt sleeves shovelling a lot of other men into a fiery furnace. There were times when I could have happily shovelled Reginald in with them. The conversation in the teashop later regularly followed the same pattern.

'Would you like a crumpet, dear?'

'Oh, I couldn't really. I'm not the least little bit hungry.' Liar.

'I'm sure you could eat just one little one if you tried.'

'Well if you insist, perhaps just one.'

We often had to wait ten minutes for the crumpet to arrive and another ten minutes before the pot of tea got there. Reginald wasn't the sort of man to have waitresses falling over themselves to serve him. When the crumpet eventually arrived I demolished it in two hungry bites thinking yearningly of the sausage sandwiches in the dirty café. Tainted or not I would have swapped the crumpet anytime for one sauce-filled mouthful.

After the crumpet we took a gentle stroll down Mansfield Road waiting for the church to open, and after church we took another gentle stroll up Mansfield Road waiting for it to be time for me to go in. Outside the lodge gates Reginald would hold my hand for a split second and look as if he might be going to kiss me, then thought better of it and we went our separate ways, he to the workhouse and me to the home taking in the scent of the wallflowers on my way there. There was never any inducement to do a slide down the railway bank. Reginald's mother had brought him up to remain upright in the teeth of temptation, and he remained faithful to her teachings.

On the day she came down from her eyrie in the North to inspect me I was on my best behaviour. Reginald had warned me that his mother disapproved of words like 'God' or any other mention of the Trinity or branches of it, so I didn't once say God, nor did I smoke while she was there. Reginald had told me she didn't approve of smoking either. She questioned me as closely as the prelim examiners had and seemed reasonably satisfied with the answers I gave her. She warned Reginald to be sure to put on his long underpants the moment the weather got cooler and off she went, leaving me to ponder over the underpants and all they implied.

When I took him home for my mother to have a look at she was delighted with him. He was exactly what she would have chosen for me, quiet, well-spoken and almost ladylike at times. She gave us her blessing before we had asked for it.

The engagement was a foregone conclusion among our mutual friends. They clubbed together to buy us a set of fish knives and forks, E.P.N.S., just as we had clubbed together to give Weldon, Davies and Baker a set of fish knives and forks when they got engaged. In return Reginald took us all to Lyons for a crumpet and a pot of tea. He at least spared us the Art Gallery.

It was when our mutual friends started planning what they were going to give us for a wedding present that panic set in. I had realized for a long time that something was lacking in the courtship. It had none of the fire that had buckled my knees behind the bathroom door, and none of the drive that made me bike all the way to Chesterfield, and certainly none of the wickedness that sent me hurtling down the railway bank hot from Eric's attentions. I would have welcomed a mixture of all three.

As the walk down the aisle with Reginald closed in on me my panic grew. I spent hours thinking up ways of telling him, his mother, my mother and all our friends that I didn't want to marry him. I even tried quarrelling with him, hoping that a quarrel might kindle some sort of flame.

'Why don't you quarrel with me for a change?' I asked him one Sunday evening as we were coming out of church. He looked at me as if I had taken leave of my senses. Reginald had never had a cross word with anybody in his life.

'Pardon,' he said, refusing to believe his ears. I repeated the suggestion.

'But my dear girl, what is there to quarrel about?' he asked, puzzled. I obviously had to employ different tactics from that if I wanted to get rid of him. I tried being late for dates but that didn't work either; he simply stood about waiting patiently until I turned up. His mother made her side of it easier for me. She came back to have another look at me and I did all the things she disapproved of. I chain-smoked all the time, and said 'God' as often as I could get it in. She went away convinced that I was not the girl for her Reginald, but I still had him and my mother to convince. I took Weldon, Davies, Baker and the Irish girl into my confidence but though they sympathized they had no advice to offer me. I became more and more depressed. I thought of running away but I had nowhere to run. I thought of Lysol, then I remembered Strickland's face when we found her and thought again. I tried drowning myself in the bath, but the moment the water got anywhere near my mouth I panicked and took the plug out. I thought of morphia, but all that dissolving the tablet in a teaspoon over the bunsen burner put me off. There seemed nothing left for me but to marry Reginald. Then Baker's brother came along and solved all my most immediate problems for me. Though he created a lot of new ones in their place.

Baker's brother was a sailor and as dashing as Eric had been, and just as wicked. When he came home on leave he took us all to the Kardomah and treated us to a cup of coffee and a slice of fruit cake. His fruit cake was a lot tastier than Reginald's crumpet, and when he asked Baker to ask me if I would go to the pictures with him I didn't hesitate. We walked to the pictures through the snow, singing as we walked.

'I'm looking for an angel,' he bellowed.

'But angels are so few,' I bawled. When we got as far as 'I'll string along with you' I had made up my mind.

The 'Dear Reginald' letter I wrote was very sad. I told him I had long ago realized I was not good enough for him, I stressed how heartbroken I was and I concluded by wishing him a speedy recovery from the anguish I was causing him. Six months later he married a Sister who would make a splendid Matron for the workhouse he was planning to be Master of and they moved up north to be nearer his mother. Where she would no doubt keep an eagle eye on them both.

I wrote a similar letter to my mother but reversed the situation. I told her how Reginald had said I was not good enough for him, I stressed how heartbroken I was and concluded by wishing myself a speedy recovery from the anguish he was causing me. She sent me a postal order for five shillings, reminded me that there were as many fish in the sea as ever came out of it and told me to keep smiling – which I did.

I hung on to the engagement ring and the fish knives and forks and after allowing a decent time to elapse I pawned the lot and we all went and had a slap-up meal in the small dirty café that had sprung up where the other one used to be.

Chapter Seventeen

WORKING ON THE Children's ward was never the joy we hoped it would be. Any thoughts we may have had of it being three months of cuddling babies and playing with toddlers were soon destroyed. They were destroyed even before we got there. 'You're bloody welcome to it,' said the Irish girl when Davies and I saw our names down for the Children's Block. The Irish girl said 'bloody' a lot. Once when she had just come from church we asked her how she could go to church and come back swearing as much as ever. She gave the question her earnest attention for a minute then came up with the logical answer. 'And did it never occur to the one of you how much worse I might have been swearing if I hadn't just been to church?' After that the word 'hypocrite' sprang to mind less readily when we thought of her beads and her swearing.

'You'll hate every minute of it on the Children's Block,' she went on. 'The sister's hardly ever there.

When she's off she's off, and when she's on she's off somewhere drinking tea with the housemen.'

'Well at least she won't be nagging us,' said Davies, hopefully.

'Maybe she won't, but the staff-nurse will,' replied the Irish girl. 'She's a bloody shocker.' Our blood froze. A shocker of a staff-nurse could often be worse than a shocker of a sister. We thanked the Irish girl for her words of encouragement and went across to the Children's Block.

We had not been misinformed. In place of the moody, exacting and often downright horrible sister we had come to know and expect we now had a staff-nurse who was all these things with a few of her own qualities thrown in, none of them nice. She was savage with us and unkind to the children. When she was about they stopped whatever they were doing, whether it was laughing, crying, talking or playing, and lay to attention in their beds waiting for her to jump on them. They never had to wait long.

'Billy Smith.'

'Yes, Nurse?'

'Why is your comic lying on the floor instead of on your locker?'

'Please, Nurse, I dropped it.'

'Then get straight out of bed and pick it up.'

'Yes, Nurse.'

'Billy Smith.'

'Yes, Nurse?'

'What are you doing out of bed?'

'Please, Nurse, you told me—'

'How dare you argue with me. Get back into that bed at once.'

'Yes, Nurse.' And we would look the other way and wait until the staff-nurse had gone before we cuddled the hurt child to make him feel wanted again. It took a lot of courage to stand up to our seniors, especially anyone as senior as a staff-nurse. Davies tried it once and a lot of good it did her.

'Nurse Davies.'

'Yes, Nurse.'

'For God's sake, tie that child's hands behind its back and stop it scratching its spots.' Davies looked at the spotty child and at the staff-nurse.

'But, Nurse,' she said, 'if I put a pair of mittens on her like we did on the others she won't be able to scratch her spots.' The staff-nurse nearly had a fit.

'Are you questioning my authority?' she screamed.

'Yes, Nurse,' said Davies. I looked from one to the other with my mouth open. And especially at Davies. I would never have thought she was capable of such mutiny. She stood her ground and the staff-nurse stood hers. The staff-nurse won on points. She had technical advantages over Davies. 'Go to the Matron at once,' she ordered, beside herself with rage. 'Don't wait till the morning, go now and tell her that you have refused to obey my command.' Then she turned to me. 'Tie that child's hands behind its back and let me hear no more about it.' And I did. The fact that I tied them so loosely that the child would hardly notice they were tied at all was no excuse for my cowardice. I was no heroine.

When Davies went to the office the Matron was very harsh with her.

'How dare you disobey your seniors?' she said cuttingly.

'But, Matron—' began Davies. The Matron raised her hand.

'I will not have my nurses being insubordinate to their seniors.'

'But, Matron—' Davies tried again. Again the Matron held up her hand.

'Silence, Nurse, you will not improve things by defying me as well. A staff-nurse is in sole charge of the ward during the sister's absence and must be given respect and obedience. Kindly remember that in future.'

'But, Matron—' struggled Davies, determined to be heard, 'the child was ill and lonely and her spots were itching. All I wanted to do was to try and make her feel a little more comfortable and a bit happier.' The Matron sat for a moment weighing up this piece of fresh evidence then she delivered her verdict and it went against Davies.

'Whether a child is ill or not, Nurse, is no excuse for pampering it. You must learn to draw the line between kindness and pampering. Firmness is the key when we are dealing with the young and you would do well to remember it. And furthermore, if you persist in this belligerent behaviour I shall have no alternative but to mention it in your hospital report which could label you as a troublemaker for the rest of your career. We do not want this to happen, do we, Nurse?'

'No, Matron. Thank you, Matron,' said Davies and crawled out of the office.

She was very upset when she told us about it afterwards.

'Do there have to be bruises before anybody will believe that children get hurt?' she asked us bitterly. 'Somebody ought to tell the Matron that bruises don't always show.' I kept quiet. I wasn't going to be the one to tell her. But I knew that Davies was right. The children on that particular children's ward must have been a mass of bruises beneath the surface where the staff-nurse had got at them.

If summers were more summery in those days, and winters more wintry, then illness was certainly iller. Children were brought in doomed to die from simple things which soon would cause no more inconvenience than a day or two off school. Many of the things they died of were later to become so rare as to warrant a mention in the press when they did occur. The advent of antibiotics shifted the balance of power from nursing as we knew it to a quick jab with a needle and it was all over. They cured in days things it took us weeks to work on with ice-packs, hot fomentations and pneumonia jackets. Disease went according to the text books of the time, and if a child got better when the book said it wouldn't, we marvelled at it and talked about it in the mess-room.

'Here, guess what, you know that baby I was specialling, the one that was going to die?' Which one when there were so many of them going to die?

'You mean the one with diphtheria that had to have the trachy the other night?' They were having trachys all the time, day and night.

'That's the one, well guess what, it went home today.'

'It didn't.' Why should it when so many didn't?

'It did.'

'My God.' We were never as surprised when they died as we were when they lived. Even the parents were taken aback when we told them their child was getting better. Diphtheria was a killer, whooping cough was a killer, ear infections that started out being simple ear infections quickly became killers, tuberculosis was killing or crippling all the time. We made tiny pneumonia jackets and tiny cotton-wool shrouds by the dozen and seldom had any in stock. However reluctant we had been before to bleed for our patients none of us could help a little bleeding on the children's wards. We bled as much for the parents as we did for the patients.

'He won't die will he, Nurse? He's all we've got,' they pleaded as they handed over their steaming hot, shivering little mite, expecting miracles.

'Of course he won't,' we promised them, already wondering what we were going to say to them when he died, having failed to work miracles.

'We never had enough money to feed him properly,' said the mother guiltily when she delivered her rickety baby to us. Nor the other six at home either.

'Their mother's in the Sanatorium with consumption,' explained the father trying to hide his relief at being able to deposit his consumptive children on us. The wards were full of rickety children, under-nourished children, tubercular children and dying children. We splinted their limbs, straightened their spines, forced milk into them, choked them with Dr Dean's garlic and still they died. Even the fresh air on the ice-cold verandahs did nothing to save their lives.

When we were not busy with splints, spinal jackets and pneumonia jackets we shaved pathetic little heads. Scabies, impetigo, ringworm and lice were occupational hazards among school children and their younger brothers and sisters. We nitted them, sulphur-bathed them, and painted their ringworms with iodine. When the staff-nurse was out of the way and it was safe to laugh they laughed at each other's bald heads, forgetting that they were as bald as coots themselves.

None of the children appreciated the baths we gave them, whether they were bran baths, starch baths or just plain soap-and-water baths. The total immersion we subjected them to was something outside their experience. They kicked and screamed and fought to avoid getting involved in the vendetta we waged against them, which they took to be a personal insult. We approached them armed to the teeth with towels, flannels and soap. They might just as well have been guns for the terror they struck in the children's minds.

'Gerraway. I's not going in that water again today. I wen' in it yesterday.' Bang.

'Oh yes you are, my lad, in you go.' Crash.

'Lemme out it's wet.' Splosh.

'Of course it's not. Don't be silly.' Splash.

'Lemme out it's 'ot.' Thrash.

'You stay just where you are.'

'Lemme out.' When the bathing was finally over we were as wet as they were. Most of them went home a lot cleaner than when they came in.

'Don't I look lovely?' said one little girl, seeing her pink skin for the first time in her life, after we had scraped off the last of the scaly scabs.

'No you don't. You look bloody soppy,' said her four-year-old brother contemptuously. 'I liked you best when you was mucky.' The baby of the family said nothing. He sat in his cot too flea-bitten and scabby to want to talk.

When two children were brought in to us one day they were neither nitty nor scabby. They were clean and neat and had perfect manners. The boy was very protective towards his younger sister. They had been in several days when one of the other children turned to them after visiting time.

'Our mam just told me anty that your mam's been hung for killing somebody.' There was a dreadful silence round about and the boy got out of bed and put his arm round his sister. It was the first either of them had heard about it but they didn't argue. Up to then they had thought their mam had gone to heaven to be with Jesus. It took us a long time to convince them that she had, in spite of what the other children were saying about her. I don't think we ever really managed it. Though maybe it wasn't too far from the truth. The grandmother told us her daughter had been a wonderful mother and the children were living proof of that, which may have helped her when she reached the Gates.

Visiting days on the children's wards were awful. They were on Wednesdays and Saturdays, and not on

Sundays like all other wards. This meant that more mums turned up than dads. Dads had better things to do on Saturday afternoon than sit beside a cot while the child in it screamed to be taken out of it. The tumult on the Notts Forest home ground was more attractive than our noisy jungle could ever be.

Not all the children screamed at first. Most of them hadn't seen their mother for a week, as most of the mothers went out to work, and a week was a long time. Grannies came on Wednesday but that wasn't the same, they only came to have a chat with the other grannies that turned up. Instead of being transported with delight at the sudden appearance of their mothers, the children either screamed with fury at being so mercilessly dumped on strangers, or maintained a sullen silence and refused to recognize their visitor. Just when they were beginning to have a dim recollection, it was time for the mother to go and the child raised its voice in protest at her going. Those who had never stopped screaming found fresh voice to scream louder and the few who really had enjoyed visiting day became desolate when it was over and joined in the chorus. Mothers said their farewells and went, only to come back a second or two later to say them again. The children wailed even louder and the mothers went off weeping. Just when things were beginning to settle down a bit of the mothers would decide to have another quick peep through the screens we had put at the door and every child in the ward saw her and resented the fact that it wasn't their mother, and voiced their resentment. Visiting day was one of the few times we were grateful for the staff-nurse's intervention. With one sharp command she was able to quell the cacophony that had us beaten.

When the last runny nose had been blown and the last choking sob stemmed we looked at each other and thanked heaven that visiting day was only twice a week and for only an hour at a time. If we could have had our way it would have been stopped altogether. We all agreed that it did more harm than good. None of us could have foreseen a time when visiting day would be all day and every day, and night as well if an anxious mother wanted it that way.

Chapter Eighteen

Davies's fears of catching TB when she went on Female Sanatorium were mild in comparison to the terror we felt when we were put on Female Venereal. None of us went on Male Venereal. Only the male nurses went on there. They had a Mister instead of a Sister in charge of them and they lived in mortal fear of him. He was an ex-Army nurse and ran his ward with military precision. He had inspections in the mornings and parades at night, and would have welcomed a detention room if the authorities had allowed it. The patients stood before him stark naked while he examined them for further erosions of the disease they were in for. He picked up what was usually the most affected portion with a pair of forceps and dropped it with disgust when he saw the early treatment they had had the day before had done little to stop the rot. He was not disgusted with the patient; he was only disgusted with the failure of the treatment. None of us were disgusted with the patients; we left that to their own consciences.

'My God,' said the Irish girl as we trailed across to Female Venereal. 'Just think of it, bloody VD' We thought of it in silence for the next few yards. Both of us could picture the coloured plates in the text books which gave a vivid impression of the disease in its more advanced stage. They were horrifying.

'Never mind,' I said, trying to console the Irish girl. 'The sister on there's Irish so that ought to make things a bit easier for you, at least she'll let you go to Mass when you want.' Some of the Church of England sisters were very difficult about letting the Irish nurses go to Mass. She refused to be comforted.

'Fat lot of use Mass will be when I'm eaten away with syphy.'

We fell silent again imagining the worst.

The building we were walking to stood on its own in a remote part of the hospital grounds. It was divided off into separate units, and was almost a small hospital in itself. There was a nursery, a maternity block, a children's ward, two female wards and a chronic unit. The sister in charge of it was not only Irish, she was an Irish saint. She spent as much of her time trying to save the patients' souls as she spent trying to save their bodies. In both cases some of it worked and a lot of it didn't. She had a gentle manner and a nun-like face. As far as we could discover she had only one weakness. That was 'Garth' in the *Daily Mirror*. Garth was a great hefty he-man in one of the comic strips. The sister on Female Venereal never missed a trick of his. Even on her days off we had to take him up to her room with the breakfast tray the sisters were allowed in bed when they were off. When she went on holiday we had to cut him out of the paper and save him for her until she came back. Apparently they didn't have a Garth in Ireland. He seemed to satisfy her every instinct, feminine, maternal and any baser ones she may have nurtured in her bosom. Whatever her dreams Garth was the answer to them.

The first thing she did when we reported on duty was take us in the office and give us a little talk. She reminded us that her ward had several different features from other wards we had worked on. She told us that our safety depended on us keeping strictly to the rules of hygiene as we had been taught to do in the lecture room. Unless we did, she said, she would not be answerable for the consequences.

'There, what did I tell you?' whispered the Irish girl savagely. 'We'll all go off here riddled.'

'Were you wishing to say something, Nurse?' inquired the sister.

'No, Sister. Thank you, Sister,' said the Irish girl.

'Then kindly keep quiet and listen to what I am telling you.' The Irish girl kept quiet and listened. The sister went on.

'Many of the patients on this ward are victims of their own folly but others are victims of cruel circumstances. It is not for us to form opinions or pass judgement, it is for us to nurse each one with the same impartial kindness. It will, however, be from the example we set that they may come to see the error of their ways, if error there is.' We doubted it. Our ways were too erratic for anyone to take example from. We left that part of it to the sister and contented ourselves with doing everything for the patients on Female Venereal that we would have done for the patients anywhere else, but with a lot more hand-scrubbing in between. And changed our knickers twice a week instead of once.

The doctor who visited the ward was a tower of strength. He was elderly and aristocratic and a bachelor. We suspected he was a little in love with the sister but he had too much competition in the shape of Garth.

'Will we catch it?' the Irish girl asked him one day when she suspected she'd got it.

'Not if you're careful,' he told her.

'And what if we're not?' she asked.

'Then you'll rot like the patients are doing,' he told her cheerfully. His answer did the Irish girl a lot of good and me as well.

'I've really got it this time,' I groaned to Baker for the tenth time in a week.

'Where?' she said, edging away. She had done her stint on Female Venereal and had escaped unscathed; she had no intention of getting contaminated by me.

'Here,' I said, showing her an almost invisible pimple on my bottom.

'It's a pimple,' she said.

'It's a syphilitic sore,' I said. She had another look at it.

'My God, you're right,' she said, and I rushed off in a panic to show the doctor my bottom. It was a pimple but it took him a long time to convince me.

Again, working on the Children's ward was not a happy experience. The babies and toddlers were all suffering too much from the sins of their fathers – or mothers. When the fathers and the mothers came to visit them we tried to remember sister's warnings and not look down our noses too much, but it was hard not to sometimes, especially when the children were sadly afflicted.

One mother who came to the nursery didn't even try not to look down her nose at us. She was young and beautiful. She had two children who were young and beautiful as well. Unfortunately they would both be blind before they got much older. Every Saturday after-noon their mother came to see them laden with parcels that had been sent specially from a famous London store. She rolled up in a limousine and a chauffeur jumped out to open the door for her and help her with the parcels. He was careful when he shut the car door not to get her furs jammed. She was clearly at the very summit of her profession. None of us had reached the summit of our profession and even when we did there would be no limousine and no chauffeur to open doors for us. We would still be struggling with our own parcels, for the most part, from Woolworth's.

One of the nurses who knew all about the young woman told us she had worked very hard to get where she was.

'Her mother and her grandmother are ever so proud of her,' the nurse said, a little proudly.

'Why are they?' we asked.

'Well, because of the way she has worked her way up. They were just common prostitutes and never got further than Long Row and Slab Square.' Both were the local Piccadilly Circus and both were famed for their brisk turnover in prostitutes.

'How far has she worked her way up?' we asked, fascinated.

'Well, you know you-know-who?' We nodded. We didn't exactly know him but we'd read a lot about him in the gossip columns.

'She happens to be his mistress,' said our informant and waited for our reactions. We gasped. We knew enough about you-know-who to know that to work your way up any higher than him, it would have to be royalty.

After that we did a little door opening ourselves when the children's mother arrived; we even stooped to pick up any parcels she dropped on the way to the nursery. We hoped a little of her fame might have brushed off onto us. It didn't. Whenever she swept past us our caps seemed grubbier, our shoes sloppier and our black woollen stockings holier. The sister had a different outlook which she voiced one day.

'If I thought the time would come when that innocent child would grow up to follow her mother's profession I would rather see her dead.' Strong words but we knew that she meant all she said, and though none of us was saintly enough to see things the way she saw them, her comments at least put things back in perspective for us. Instead of envying the mother her riches we started thinking of the children more, and pitying them. We left the parcels for the chauffeur to pick up. No doubt he got well paid for his trouble.

The Maternity ward was not a happy place to work in either. Far too many babies were born there less than perfect. The only bit of light relief we got was towards the end of every delivery when the sister would gather every member of her staff together round the bed and just as the tiny head – or rump – was making its appearance she would close her eyes tightly and in a loud voice entreat us: 'Pray, Nurses, pray.' As far as I knew none of us ever prayed and the baby got born or didn't get born the same as if we had. Maybe the sister's prayers were enough to ensure its safe delivery.

There were tragedies on the women's wards that matched the tragedies on the children's wards. As we had been warned by sister on our first day, some were in through their own foolishness but others were there through no fault of their own. One such patient was brought in by her husband on a day arranged by their own doctor, who had not had the courage to tell them why he was sending the woman in to us. They were an ordinary middle-class couple who had lived an ordinary middle-class life until the husband strayed from the path of virtue just once, with terrible consequences. It was only when he looked through the office window and realized where the ward was located that he recognized it for what it was and knew why he was bringing his wife there. It took us longer to treat him for shock than it took to comfort the wife. He had guilt to live with; she had only pain and sorrow. He lived longer with his guilt than she had to live with her sorrow.

The Chronic ward was something we all preferred to forget. There was no joy for anybody on there. It was a place where the sins of the past – if sins there had been – were forgotten, but the price for them was still being paid, and in full. We were all glad when our stint there was finished.

The part of the building most of us enjoyed working on was the ward where the court cases were sent to be treated and possibly, if only temporarily, cured. Here the girls were mostly young and mostly prostitutes, and mostly unrepentant prostitutes. None of them seemed to mind being where they were and none of them seemed to mind being what they were. Contrary to the wishful thinking of the more vociferous evangelical movements, they showed no signs of wanting to be saved. They were doing very nicely as they were, thank you very much. And listening to the story of their life we couldn't help thinking that they were doing a lot better than we were.

'Why do you do it?' we asked them, earnestly wanting to know.

'Why do you do what you're doing?' they countered.

'I suppose because we want to,' we said, doubtfully if it had been a bad day.

'Yes. Well then, that's why we do what we are doing,' they told us. We were forced to the conclusion that sin couldn't be as wicked as we were brought up to believe it was, and basically sinners weren't so very different from us. Most of the girls were financially better off than we were and didn't hesitate to throw scorn on us for choosing a profession that demanded such long hours.

'Catch me working from seven o'clock in the morning to nine at night,' said Laura, who was nearing the top of her profession but had still a long way to go before she reached the limousine and chauffeur stage. 'I only do an hour or two in the afternoon and a bit in the evening.'

'What do you do the rest of the day?' we asked her as she lolled in the sluice watching us working.

'Oh, this and that,' she said. 'I usually get up about nine, unless I've had a late client, then I take the poodle for a walk in the arboretum, pop in to the clinic for a chat to the doctors and a quick check-up, see a couple of customers in the afternoon then get taken out for dinner or something in the evening.' She made it all sound so easy that we began to wonder who was right, she and the rest of our girls or the evangelists and us. We were still wondering even when the police brought her back for further treatment.

One of the regulars on the probation block was Phyllis. She looked a bit like Bertha in the lecture room. She was blonde and buxom and looked as if she had been practised on for quite a while. She wasn't in the same professional stratum as Laura. She had progressed no further than Long Row and was always getting picked up and sent in to us. She was a good cook and when she came in she usually brought little dainties with her so that we could have a celebration when the sister's back was turned. We never minded eating her cooking, we knew she was scrupulously clean, at least where it showed.

If Pickford had been a headache to the sister-tutor, Phyllis was an even bigger headache to the sister on Female Venereal. Opposite the ward a gang of workmen were laying the foundations for a new building. One morning the foreman came over with his cap in his hand and a worried look on his face. The worried look was even more worried when he was confronted by the sister and her saintly face. He hadn't expected to have to deal with a saint, however prepared he was to meet angels. It took him a long time to start off.

'Can I help you?' said the sister. He twiddled his cap and coughed.

'Well, Miss. I hardly like to mention it,' he said at last. 'Please do,' begged the sister. He made a determined effort and proceeded.

'Well, it's like this 'ere, Miss. There's a young woman on this ward.' He stopped.

'Yes?' pressed the sister.

'Well, Miss, this young woman you've got on 'ere comes across to the building site and stops the men from working. I wish you could see your way clear to keeping her locked up at least until we've laid the foundations. We'll never get the place finished at this rate.'

The sister looked at him kindly.

'Ah yes, you mean Phyllis,' she said. The man put his cap on again.

'I don't know what she's called, Miss. All I know is that she's a right nuisance across there. The men must spend a fortune on her, begging your pardon, Miss.' Then he went.

Phyllis was warned not to go to the building site again so she spent her days walking up and down the verandah in full view of the men, with her dressing gown flapping open showing a lot of leg, and a bit more besides sometimes. The men spent hours gazing wistfully at her, remembering happier times.

We suffered as much as they did from the ban. While Phyllis was keeping them busy in their meal-breaks, she was in the money and could afford to buy us little luxuries like a packet of cigarettes when our funds were low. It never bothered us that we were smoking on her immoral earnings; we were only too glad to get the cigarettes never mind how they had been come by. Phyllis was as generous to us as she was to the men. Male Venereal had more than its usual quota of building-site workers for early treatment that year.

On Wednesday afternoons the sister held a little prayer meeting in her office. All the girls were rounded up and made to attend, and as many of us as could be spared from our duties. The meetings were a tremendous success. While the sister stood with her eyes shut praying for their souls, the girls were making plans for getting them damned. The plans were usually detailed descriptions of their last escape improved upon to make their next escape more difficult to track down. They were always escaping. Whenever one of them nipped through a lavatory window and scrambled up the railway bank for an hour or two's freedom, apart from informing the police there was never too much panic. We all knew they would come back when their hunger was satisfied, however much damage they caused while they were satisfying it. Neither did we waste too much sympathy on their victims. If one of them should find himself standing in front of Mister-with-his-forceps, it was a risk they had to take.

When Laura went home she invited me round to her flat one day. It was situated in the best end of the town and was very opulent. It was the most opulent place I had ever been in in my life, except when we went to the pictures. There was a day-bed in it with red plush coverings with pom-poms on which matched the red plush curtains with pom-poms at the windows. Even the lavatory seat had a plush cover on it. I was overawed by it all. I was even more overawed by Laura's clothes. She wore a flowing tea gown sort of thing with lace all over it. I felt very dowdy in comparison. The poodle greeted me warmly. He was used to meeting strangers. His name was Fifi-Fifi, but he was clearly a boy.

After Laura had shown me round the flat we sat on the day-bed and I showed her how to knit. We had just got round to purling when the doorbell rang. Laura shoved the knitting under a chair, bustled me out of the back door and I never went there again.

When I saw her in Long Row a week or two later she told me that the poodle had eaten the knitting while she was busily engaged on the day-bed and was still going about with an agonized expression on its face and strands of blue wool dangling from its bottom. She said she had given up trying to learn how to knit and had taken up crosswords instead; they were easier to discard when the doorbell rang.

The girls all loved the aristocratic old doctor and flirted with him whenever he did a round. He seemed to enjoy their flirting and never put them down either by word or look. He treated them with the same courtesy as he treated us and every other woman. Whether he had strong feelings about the way they earned their living, he never showed it and they respected him for treating them as women, neither scarlet nor wicked.

In the winter when the weather was at its worst he went round the wards enveloped in a fur coat and wearing a pair of sheepskin gloves that reached almost up to his elbows. While he was chatting to the girls a drop would gather on the end of his nose and quiver there until it seemed certain that it would fall on the case sheet he was examining. The girls watched it with bated breath. At the precise moment that it was ready to detach itself from his nose he scooped it up delicately with his thumb and completed the operation with a sweeping movement from thumb to wrist. There was a permanent black mark on his right glove that got blacker as the years went by. He knew perfectly well the fascination the drop on his nose held for the girls, and as he rescued it from its downward flight, he would grin at them mischievously. 'Thought I'd missed it that time, didn't you?' he'd say, and they would start to watch the next drop gather.

Just before we were due to come off Female Venereal the Irish girl killed a patient just by saying a kind word to her, or so she persuaded herself into believing for a long time.

The patient was the woman who had her husband to thank for her being on the ward at all. Soon after she was brought in it was discovered that as well as the disease she officially came in with she had raging tuberculosis of both lungs and she was put into a cubicle on her own. Her husband visited her as often as he was allowed to, not just to make amends for the damage he had done but because he loved her very dearly. She had forgiven him long before he was able to forgive himself.

We were fond of them both, the wife for her loyalty to her husband and him because, in spite of his single slide from the straight and narrow, we knew he was basically a good man and as much a victim of cruel circumstance as she was. We went out of our way to give him a cup of tea whenever he came. A cup of tea is a nurse's way of showing favouritism, either to a patient or to a visitor.

One morning when the Irish girl stood in the cubicle arranging the roses the husband had brought the night before, she stopped messing about with the flowers and turned to the woman in the bed.

'Sure and it's a lovely husband you've got, Mrs Moore,' she said.

'Well, I think so, Nurse,' said Mrs Moore, smiling gratefully.

'Can I have him when you've finished with him?' asked the Irish girl.

'You'll have to wait a long time, I hope,' said the woman, laughing. She laughed too much and one of her damaged lungs collapsed under the strain and she died at once.

What with that, and winning all the money, the Irish girl never slept properly again. We were all glad when she had passed her finals and was able to go ahead with her plans for America. She might have been happier being a nun instead. She came back to see us once and told us that America wasn't all it was cracked up to be. She said she wouldn't mind it so much if they spoke

English. She had a lot of trouble understanding what they were talking about.

War had broken out when she came back, and someone remarked at the plight of the poor little birds being buffeted about with bombs and things. The Irish girl reminded the speaker that there had been a gap of more than twenty years since the last war. 'They've had a bloody long rest,' she said unfeelingly.

Chapter Nineteen

AND SUDDENLY WE were within weeks of sitting for our finals. As the day loomed nearer any hopes we may have had of ever becoming State Registered Nurses ebbed and flowed at a tremendous rate. One minute we were looking old and haggard as we thought of the misspent hours of our three years' training, courting when we should have been cramming our heads with knowledge and biking to Newstead when we should have been conserving our energies for working all night and studying all day: the next we shed a few years again while we allowed ourselves to hope that someday – who knew – we might even end up a sister at some backwater of a hospital where they didn't mind too much about the black marks on our hospital report.

When the tide was running in our favour and we were able to see ourselves as bullying staff-nurses instead of merely being bullying third-year nurses we closeted ourselves in our rooms and tried on our bows.

This had to be done with the utmost secrecy. The secrecy was so that none of our friends could accuse us of being big-headed enough to assume we might get our bows, and so that we didn't tempt fate into snatching them from us at the last minute.

Like calling the dining-room the mess-room, 'getting our bows' was the hospital's own special way of saying we had passed our finals. Getting our bows meant that instead of clamping our caps to our heads with Kirby grips as we had done for the past three years, we were entitled to tie them on with lengths of tape with delicate lacy bows at the ends. The bows were tied beneath our chin – or chins, according to the amount of weight we carried. We spent hours of our days off choosing the lace and sewing it onto the tape, not to mention the hours we stood in front of a mirror practising tying the bows. However much we practised we ended up looking much the same as we had done while we were probationers: the born nurses with their bows looking like bows and always in the right place, and the nursing-thrust-upon-them ones managing to get them under one ear or untied altogether. Passing our finals didn't turn us automatically into born nurses, but what it did do was send our salary leaping from twenty-two pounds a year to twenty-five. We built fantastic castles in the air, using the extra three pounds as bricks. The mind boggled at earning as much as twenty-five pounds a year and just for doing everything.

Sister-tutor lost a lot of weight, and possibly a little heart as well, drumming things into us at the last minute which we should have known perfectly well without any extra drumming. Later, she lost so much weight that they took her to the theatre to find out where it had gone and brought her back to the ward lighter by yet another few pounds. She stuck her chin up in bed and behaved with the same gentlewomanly pride she had reminded us of when we irritated her with our juvenile giggling in the lecture room.

The male nurses came on duty in the morning rough-cheeked with sitting up half the night studying and not having time to get a proper shave. Though they wouldn't have any bows to show for their three years' hard labour it was as important to them as it was to us that they should pass their finals and go on to be misters of Male Venereals and Male Sanatoriums some-where else.

Weldon, Baker and Davies laid aside the chair-back covers and the hand towels they were embroidering with 'His' and 'Hers' on them and tried to catch up on things they had missed while they were planning what to dress the bridesmaids in. Dr Collins and Harry took up cycling to sublimate their unquenched passions.

The Irish girl threw herself into a frenzy of surgery

and medicine, not just to forget what Mrs Moore had looked like when she died, but in order to be able to boast to the Americans that she was a State Registered Nurse – British style – when she got over there. Not that they were particularly impressed; they did things differently in America.

I had a last splendid row with Baker's brother which came just in time for me to curl up among the springs in the sitting-room and read up hernias and brush up my mammary glands. Baker's brother was not a bit like Reginald. He had never needed any invitation to quarrel, he was doing it all the time. This set me off and together we had some right royal fights. I missed his wars far more than I missed Reginald's peace.

And all the time life was going on in the wards as if we had nothing more to worry about than looking after patients.

The Irish girl went into the theatre on the next change day and came out of it bitterly disappointed. She had expected a lot more from it.

'All that bloody nonsense you see on the pictures,' she grumbled. 'Nurses and doctors gazing at each other and falling in love while they are tearing somebody's inside out, it ought to be banned. All I ever do in the theatre is wash walls down and empty buckets.' We knew how she felt. We had all been sadly let down the first time we went in the theatre. We went in heady with excitement and came out bored to tears by the surgeon's detailed account of the size of the salmon he had caught in Scotland somewhere. He brought us a bit once, but I didn't care much for it, I preferred a bit of best red tinned any time. The nearest most of us got to handling the instruments was when we had to clean them when it was all over. The Irish girl had a right to feel aggrieved. There must be a lot of young girls who decide to be a nurse on the strength of the passionate encounters across an operating table which she has read about or seen on the films. No mention is ever made of the hard work that goes into it before a trolley is laid up, and the even harder work that is left to be done after the patient has been wheeled away.

Davies came off the terminal wards looking tired and sad. 'My God,' she burst out one day, when we were puffing our lives away in the library. 'What are we supposed to say to them when they ask?'

'When who asks what?' we asked.

'When the patients on the terminal wards ask us why they have to die?' We had no answers to questions like that. Even the Irish girl, with all her beads and her statues, kept quiet, not caring to be drawn into such a ticklish discussion. It was Baker who did her best to come up with a solution.

'Tell them to look it up in the Bible,' she said, as though offering them a text book for nurses.

'Don't be silly. They want real answers,' said Davies, turning down the offer.

The priests and parsons who visited the wards were asked the same question. Their answers were as inconclusive as Baker's.

'Why do I have to die?' asked the dying mothers.

'Because it is the Lord's Will, me dear.' Not enough.

'But why me?'

'He knows best.' Not many believed that he did.

'Who will feed the children when I'm gone?' asked the dying fathers.

'Their Heavenly Father, my son.'

'And buy their shoes?' Deadlock.

One of the visiting priests brought a little light relief to the wards every morning. He arrived in his tatty cassock and stained old biretta and stood at the ward door and looked around. Then, without a word of warning he went behind every set of screens that were there for whatever purpose and asked the same kindly question. 'God bless you, me dear, and are we decent today?' The remark was intended to be an inquiry after their health but so often the patient wasn't decent, being engaged in something of an extremely private nature. It would have been thought the priest might have learned from his many mistakes. He never did, and continued to embarrass his flock with his invasion of their privacy until age and infirmity kept him at home in the presbytery.

Along with all the other pearls of wisdom the sister-tutor had cast at our feet she had things to say about the nursing of terminal cases.

'Never confuse "chronic" with "terminal",' she told us one day. 'The chronics are reaching the end of a long life, usually peacefully, and are often ready and willing to die: the terminals have been brought prematurely to their end and are seldom reconciled to it. They need to be nursed with this in mind.' We did our best to remember this. We bolstered them up with false promises if they were the sort that wanted to be bolstered up, and made sure that we said nothing in front of them which might destroy the façade they had put between themselves and death. We gave them large doses of sweet sticky medicine to ease their pain, and when they had had enough of the medicine they either got more pain or they died. None of this was called euthanasia; we called it 'making them comfortable'. If life was less complicated in those days, so was dying.

The chronics needed no such bolstering. They lived so long that death had lost its terrors for them. On the day that Granny Green was a hundred we propped her up, prettied her up and put her teeth in ready for the Mayor to come and cut the cake, and read the telegram from the King if everybody had got their dates right. When the party was over and the teeth safely back in their beaker the old lady sank back in her pillows with a sigh of contentment.

'Eeh, I'm right glad that lot's over, duck,' she said to Baker who was washing the jelly off her face. 'I can knock off now and get a nice long rest. I didn't like to go before and upset the arrangements, what with the Mayor coming and everything, but now he's gone, there's nothing to keep me.'

'Where do you think you'll be going?' Baker asked her.

'God knows,' replied the old lady.

'And you could be right at that,' said Baker thoughtfully.

While the grannies lived to be a hundred and kept the Mayor busy, golden boys and fever-flushed girls coughed their lives away on the Sanatorium wards, and still managed to look beautiful while they were doing it. When two brothers, not yet twenty, died within days of each other the parents blamed us and we blamed the parents. None of us thought of blaming ignorance, and somebody had to shoulder the blame for snatching two boys away so cruelly. A lot more young men were to be snatched away before they thought up ways of killing tuberculosis just as a lot of people had to die before they thought up ways of killing flies.

When the two brothers died the Irish girl stuck her nose in the air and told everybody who would listen that she had known it would happen. She was superstitious about other things as well as the devil and the little people. She firmly believed, and talked us into believing, that if red and white flowers were arranged together in a vase and put on a locker the patient in the bed at the side of the locker was doomed to die. One morning, while she was walking past Male Sanatorium, she saw a bunch of red and white flowers on the locker between the two boys' beds. She rushed in to repair the damage but she was too late, the Fates had already noticed and set their machinery in motion. After that we were doubly careful never to put red and white flowers together.

Although we were within an ace of sitting for our finals we were still not exempt from appearing before the Matron if we had done anything to warrant her disapproval. Weldon found herself in the office one morning purely for doing an act of kindness out on the street.

The Matron had decreed that none of us should go out of the main gates in uniform until we had passed our finals. She knew only too well the damage that could be done to the casualty lying on the road by someone not too sure where the proper pressure points were to be located. A nurse in uniform laid herself wide open to such a situation. It would have sounded very feeble at the inquest to confess we didn't know our brachials from our radials. As nurses we would have been expected to know.

Poor Weldon had jumped the gun a bit. She nipped out one morning without bothering to change out of uniform and just as she was passing the bus stop outside the gates a woman who was waiting for a bus slid to the pavement at her feet. There were several other people waiting for the bus. They saw the four inches of blue and white striped dress dangling below Weldon's blue gaberdine mac and immediately expected laying on of hands and miracles. Weldon had never done a miracle in the hospital let alone outside it. She told us later that she thought of things like loosening laces and unbusking corsets but though they all sounded splendid in theory, in practice there seemed to be all sorts of snags. Suddenly she thought of the chemist's shop on the corner. She dashed across the road, explained the circumstances to the chemist and dashed back again with a tiny medicine glass of sal volatile which the chemist had told her to force between the woman's teeth. When she got to the scene of the incident there was nobody there. A bus was just drawing away and the passengers, including the woman Weldon had left sprawled on the pavement, were all sitting happily on it, waving as they went.

Weldon poured the potion down the drain then ran to the chemist's shop to return the glass. Unfortunately she tripped as she was stepping off the pavement and dropped the glass which became fragmented in the gutter.

'That will be ninepence,' said the chemist, when she told him about it.

'What for?' asked Weldon.

'Sixpence for the glass and threepence for the sal volatile.'

'But nobody drank the sal volatile,' protested Weldon.

'Can't help that,' said the chemist unsympathetically. 'The medicine was taken off my premises and therefore has to be paid for, and the glass has to be accounted for to the auditors.' Big business.

'But I've got no money,' pleaded Weldon. 'Can't I bring it in on pay day?'

'We don't give credit,' said the chemist, pointing to the notice on the wall which said 'Please don't ask for credit, a refusal may give offence'.

'What are you going to do then?' asked Weldon, seeing the debtor's prison staring her in the face.

'Take your name and address,' said the chemist. And he did, and the following morning Weldon found herself in the Matron's office charged with being outside the gates in uniform before she had passed her finals and getting goods without paying for them. Both offences told heavily against her in her hospital report.

'Catch me ever rendering first aid again,' she said furiously when she got back from being at the Matron's office. 'I wouldn't tear my petticoat into strips for anybody after this.' When we had time to read, the books we read were full of touching little tales of heroines who went about tearing their petticoats into strips for binding up wounded soldiers. None of us had ever done anything like that, and after Weldon's unhappy experience we turned our head away or dodged down a side street whenever anybody looked like crumpling to a heap in front of us. There were usually plenty of people in the crowd that gathered who knew more about first aid than we did. We were too accustomed to having the proper equipment at hand, as well as a doctor or two ready to take over before we ran out of knowledge. The Matron was quite justified in saving us from a situation that could only do harm to the reputation of the hospital, and hers as well.

I also had my pre-finals fling on the corridor at ten o'clock one morning. Mine was for being stupid enough to get caught eating on the ward. I had gone three years without that particular sin being notched up against me then a moment of carelessness cost me my record.

It was my twenty-first birthday and I was on night duty. Something seemed to be called for in the way of a little celebration so I waited until night-sister had done her two o'clock round, made sure all the patients were asleep then I went into the kitchen. I concocted a trifle with some stale Ovaltine rusks, a drop of left-over custard from the ward dinners, and a scraping of jam I found beneath a layer of green mould in a pot. I stole half a grapefruit from the diabetics' diet, boiled an egg that had already been twice boiled and tore my cob loaf into hunks. I was just chiselling the top off the egg when night-sister walked in.

Oh, Dummy, where were you in my hour of need?

We shovelled the feast into the pig bin while sister pointed out to me the error of my ways. In the morning I stood in the office trying to explain to the Matron why I had fallen so far from grace so near to sitting my finals. I didn't bother to tell her about it being my birthday, she wouldn't have been interested. I simply let her go on believing that I was gluttonous, lazy, irresponsible and willing to let my patients die while I was making a pig of myself in the kitchen. I got a mark in my hospital report as black as Weldon's.

On the evening we were to sit our finals something happened which nearly stopped us from sitting for them at all.

'Let's all go out after duty and have a stroll down Long Row,' suggested Davies. 'It's no use doing any more studying, what we don't know now we'll never know.' And we did. When we bumped into Phyllis and

Laura and Laura's mother, who were also taking a gentle stroll down Long Row though for different reasons, they were delighted to see us. Laura introduced her mother to us and we saw at a glance why she hadn't done as well as Laura. She had no ambitions to get any further than Long Row. She was very nice all the same. Granny had retired by then.

'Come on, we'll buy you a cup of tea in Lyons,' said Laura, remembering it was the end of the month and we would all be broke.

'We can't stop long,' said Phyllis. 'There's a big convention on in the town and business will be brisk.' We understood and were grateful for small mercies. When we had drunk the tea and eaten the currant buns that Laura's mother paid for we stepped out onto Long Row again and stood for a moment or two having a little chat. The two policemen who came along insisted on us all accompanying them to the station and refused to listen when Phyllis tried to tell them that we had only dropped by for a chat.

'That's all right, duck. We've heard it all before,' they said, herding us into the Black Maria. It was a long time before Baker, Weldon, Davies and I could convince them we were nurses. They believed the Irish girl because one of them was Irish and they both knew the same saints. They didn't believe the rest of us because Phyllis had told one of their mates the same story once when she had run away and was loose in Nottingham. He had kindly walked her back to the hospital and had been rewarded for his kindness behind the rhododendron bushes on the drive. When he discovered she was not a nurse he got very upset and stormed into Male Venereal and demanded a blood test. It was negative but he never really forgave Phyllis after that and was more often responsible for her being sent into us than any other policeman in Nottingham. It took a lot of proof to convince them that we were birds of a different feather from Laura and her mother and Phyllis; not necessarily better, but different.

'My mam would go out of her mind if she knew I'd been run in as a prostitute,' said Davies, wiping the tears of laughter from her eyes. And so would the Matron, we thought.

After that whenever we met any of the patients from Female Venereal outside we chose somewhere a bit less conspicuous than Long Row to stand and chat to them. The police might not have been so understanding a second time.

Whether or not we passed our finals, we had completed our three years' endurance test at the hospital and none of us looked any the worse for it. The excessive amount of carbohydrate in our diet had rounded off those who were angular by nature, though with time and sterility a lot of them would go back to being angular again: and those of us who started out being well padded had gained some extra padding over the years.

In spite of the vigilance of Mary and the gate-porters, and the constant threat of the Matron's office, any of us with an urge to sin had found plenty of opportunity for sinning. Being forbidden to do things after ten o'clock at night simply meant that you did them before ten, or stood over the dustbins praying.

In three years we had learned enough to impress the ignorant and not enough to converse about to the knowledgeable. Never having enough money to dress ourselves properly we had no dress sense; never getting the chance to mix we were poor mixers. The only people we felt truly at home with were each other and the patients who were too dependent on us to find fault with us.

In the streets and on buses we mentally stripped people who claimed an acquaintance with us on the strength that we had saved their lives at some time or other. It was only by putting them into pyjamas or nightdresses we were accustomed to seeing them in that we could get a true picture of their identity. This took time, and often by the time we had placed them they had gone, taking with them an entirely false impression of our unwillingness to acknowledge them in the street. How were they to know we were having to undress them before we recognized them?

We had lived in a world where bladders, bowels, death and destruction were discussed without even a lowering of the voice, but where none of us had ever been called by our Christian names. It was not allowed. It was unprofessional to use any but our surnames when addressing each other. However friendly we were with each other most of us went right through our training without even knowing our friends' first names. The habit died hard and afterwards, when we emerged from our cloisters, we got accused of being stand-offish because of the difficulty we had in calling casual acquaintances by their first names.

We had become so used to seeing insides lying outside and vital parts not in their proper place that nothing less than a severe case of hara-kiri could move us. Headaches had to reach brain damage and the mercury in a thermometer rise to boiling point before our interest was aroused. Someone very close to me said once: 'Do I have to die before you believe I'm ill?' He exaggerated of course, but his demise, though it might have shocked me, would at least have convinced me that he was unfit for work.

When one of the men on the building site craned his neck to get a better look at Phyllis and fell off the scaffolding, breaking both legs, an arm, his skull and sundry small bones, it was thought that on top of all his other small complaints he had a perforated gastric ulcer. An X-ray quickly proved he hadn't and the Irish girl went to reassure him on the matter.

'There's no need for you to worry,' she told him comfortingly. 'Your gastric ulcer's intact.' The man with the fractured legs, arm and head felt a lot better after that, though we personally felt that he was a bit of a malingerer complaining all the time of pain in his stomach when there was no perforated gastric ulcer to show for his pains. It was not that we were hard, it was just that we had our priorities right. Whereas a perforated gastric ulcer might have killed him, all that he would be left with was a peculiar walk, one slightly maladjusted arm and some loss of memory now and then. He should have been grateful, but he wasn't. Nobody is ever really grateful for being told that things might have been worse, any more than anyone is made to feel any better by being told that millions of other people are suffering. The fact that half the world is starving doesn't keep our hands out of the bread-bin when we are hungry.

And so we came to our finals. Overworked, underpaid and understudied, and with an immunity against bleeding for anyone but ourselves.

Chapter Twenty

THE PIECE OF paper pinned on the notice board in the mess-room told us that we were to present ourselves at the voluntary hospital on the other side of the town to sit our finals. Lunch, it said, would be provided between the morning and the afternoon papers.

'Lunch,' queried Davies. 'What do they mean, lunch? I'll need a bit more than a slice or two of bread and cheese and a cup of cocoa to see me through the day.' I agreed until I remembered the fee-paying girls at the high school, then I was able to put her mind at rest. And her stomach as well.

'Lunch is what toffee-nosed people like voluntary-trained nurses call their dinner,' I told her, backed by a superior knowledge that even going to the same school as Ray Milland couldn't compete with. She thought about it for a moment.

'Then what do they call it when they go across to their room to make their beds and change their aprons and have their bread and dripping?' she asked, showing a woeful ignorance of the niceties of gracious living.

'They probably don't have anything at all then. They'd be frightened of getting fat and they'd be too stuck-up to eat anything as common as dripping. And I bet they don't call their dining-room the mess-room either.'

'Kindly step this way and indulge in a little light refreshment in the salle-a-manger,' minced Davies affectedly. We all started giggling, then thought about the finals and stopped. We started feeling sick instead.

It was a bitter cold day and we sat on the bus shivering with cold and fright. We kept having a quick look at the text book the Irish girl had brought with her. The more we looked the less we knew.

'My God,' yelped Weldon suddenly, 'suppose we get piles.' The other passengers on the bus looked round at her and raised their bottoms an inch or two off the seats, then they shuffled about looking very worried. We looked up piles in the Irish girl's text book: excision of, post-operative treatment, and complications following excision of. It was all new to us, though it shouldn't have been. We had gone into piles in the greatest depth in the lecture room, and come across quite a number on the wards; they were very painful things we knew, but that would never have satisfied an examiner.

'Gonorrhoea,' groaned Baker – 'I bet anything I get gonorrhoea. Miller told me they all got gonorrhoea last time.' Miller was one class senior to us.

The passengers on the bus looked even more worried and started shifting their seats to get well away from Baker. We thought of getting gonorrhoea and sank into even deeper gloom.

The bus driver did his best to cheer us up. He was on the same route regularly and knew a bit about nurses.

'You ought to have been outside Lyons this morning,' he said brightly, then waited for one of us to ask him why.

'Why?' asked the Irish girl just to please him, though none of us really cared.

'There was a tart upside down in the window,' said the driver, and looked hurt when nobody laughed. He shrugged his shoulders and got on with his driving and left us to our misery.

We ploughed through the morning papers. 'Prepare the patient for this,' demanded the examiners, and we painstakingly prepared the patient for something entirely different.

'State briefly what you know about these,' begged the examiners and we scraped the barrel to find something we knew about them. It was very little.

At midday we toyed with the scrap of cold meat and beetroot the voluntary hospital gave us for our dinner, which we ate in a dining-room that was neither big, bleak or noisy. There was a sideboard at one end with a lot of silver things on it, and the dining-room maids did it all; we didn't have to get up once to help ourselves. It was all very upper crust.

In the afternoon we came face to face with our inquisitors, and the voluntary hospital's equivalent of Bertha and Ernest. They both seemed to have things wrong with them that we had never heard of. We did our best.

When it was all over we climbed wearily back on the bus. The driver was waiting for us.

'Well, did you get it?' he said when he came for our fares.

'Get what?' we asked him.

'The joke, of course.'

'What joke?'

'The joke I told you this morning. The one about the tart turned upside down in the window.' And suddenly we got it, and the picture of Laura or Phyllis upside down in the cake-shop window reduced us all to helpless choking laughter. The bus driver was gratified that his joke had gone down so well in the end and he joined in the laughter. Then the rest of the passengers asked us what the joke was and we told them and they started laughing as well and soon the bus was in an uproar.

The next few weeks of waiting for the results were agonizing. We read and re-read the examination papers.

We compared notes and swapped mistakes until we had convinced ourselves than none of us could have possibly passed our finals, then we rushed up to our rooms to have a quick try-on of our bows, just in case by some enormous fluke we had managed to fool the examiners into thinking we knew more than we did.

On the morning the results were due to be posted on the notice board we got up reluctantly, dressed ourselves slowly, snapped at each other, apologized, snapped at each other again and dragged ourselves across to the mess-room.

We shouldered our way through the milling crush and stretched and strained to find something on the board that related to us, and Davies, Weldon, Baker and the Irish girl – and me as well – had all passed our finals. We tore upstairs to get our bows and none of us ate our kippers that morning.

About the Author

Brought up in Lincolnshire, Evelyn Prentis (real name Evelyn Taws) left home at eighteen to become a nurse. She later moved to London during the war, where she married and raised her family. Like so many other nurses, she went back to hospital and used any spare time she might have had bringing up her children and running her home. Born in 1915, she sadly died in 2001 at the age of eighty-five.

Evelyn published five books about her life as a nurse, of which *A Nurse in Time* is the first. The next book, *A Nurse in Action*, about nursing during the Second World War, will be republished by Ebury Press in July 2011.

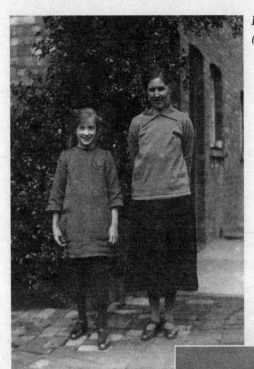

Evelyn and her
(foster) mother, 1924

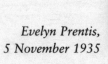

Evelyn Prentis,
5 November 1935